ATLAS

OF

VULVAR DISEASE

ATLAS
OF
VULVAR DISEASE

EDWARD J. WILKINSON

Professor
Department of Pathology
Department of Obstetrics and Gynecology
University of Florida
College of Medicine
Gainesville, Florida

I. KEITH STONE, M.D.

Associate Professor
Department of Obstetrics and Gynecology
University of Florida
College of Medicine
Gainesville Florida

*Clinical presentation with cross-reference contents
to histologic classification*

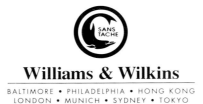

Williams & Wilkins

BALTIMORE • PHILADELPHIA • HONG KONG
LONDON • MUNICH • SYDNEY • TOKYO

A WAVERLY COMPANY

Editor: Charles W. Mitchell
Project Manager: Raymond E. Reter
Copy Editor: Molly L. Mullen
Designer: Norman W. Och
Illustration Planner: Wayne Hubbel

Accurate indications, adverse reactions, and dosage schedules for drugs are provided in this book, but it is possible that they may change. The reader is urged to review the package information data of the manufacturers of the medications mentioned.

Printed in the United States of America

Library of Congress Cataloging-in-Publication Data

Wilkinson, Edward J.
    Atlas of vulvar disease / Edward J. Wilkinson, I. Keith Stone.
    p.   cm.
    ''Clinical presentation with cross-reference contents to histologic classification.''
    Includes bibliographical references and indexes.
    ISBN 0-683-09092-5
    1. Vulva—Diseases—Atlases.   I. Stone, I. Keith.   II. Title.
    DNLM: 1. Vulvar Diseases—atlases. WP 17 W686a 1994]
RG261.W54   1994
618.1'6'00222—dc20
DNLM/DLC
for Library of Congress
                                        94-21552
                                            CIP
                             94 95 96 97 98
                1 2 3 4 5 6 7 8 9 10

This book is dedicated to physicians, nurses, and health workers committed to the care of women.

PREFACE

This atlas was written as a guide to the diagnosis, treatment, and management of vulvar disease, and is intended for use in the office or clinic. In this work is a spectrum of vulvar diseases and dermatoses that we have observed, diagnosed, treated, and managed in our vulvar clinic. Color clinical photos, as well as a corresponding histopathology, where applicable, are included. Because clinical pathologic correlation is essential for the appropriate diagnosis and treatment of vulvar disease, both clinical and histopathologic findings are presented to assist the clinician and pathologist in diagnosis and interpretation. The cases were selected as representative, and reflect a broad spectrum of clinical diseases that involve the vulva. Why an atlas on vulvar disease when there are so many good dermatologic texts covering dermatoses and neoplasms of the skin? As the reader will observe from the clinical photos herein, the expression of dermatoses, inflammatory disorders and neoplasms can be quite difficult to interpret on the vulva. The reasons for this are partially related to general lack of documentation of vulvar disorders in dermatologic texts, as well as the fact that the vulva has keratinized and nonkeratinized epithelium, hairy and nonhairy skin, and a variety of specialized glands, as well as immediate proximity to the urethra and anus. A chapter on Anatomy of the Vulva is included to address these issues.

This is provided to assist in diagnosis and classification. Line drawings of the vulva are provided to identify the topography of the vulva and to document the location of vulvar lesions when observed. A representative vulva clinic form, with attached diagrams of the vulva, is included to provide a guideline for the readers to develop their own useful working form. A listing of definitions of relevant dermatologic terms used within the work is also included.

Specific therapy is discussed within each section, in addition to the clinical color photos documenting appearance and applicable histopathology. When numerous therapeutic options are available, they are presented as progressive therapeutic options. They are presented in this manner to serve as a guide to the development of a therapeutic plan for the patient. Because many diseases of the vulva require long-term management, progressive therapeutic options can offer alternatives when a given approach fails or does not continue to be effective.

Tables on the classification of vulvar diseases, as well as on sexually transmitted diseases and vesiculobullous diseases of the vulva, are included to assist in differential diagnosis.

ACKNOWLEDGMENT

The authors acknowledge their colleagues who have assisted in the diagnoses and treatment or referred biopsies of patients discussed in this work. We also acknowledge our deceased colleague, Dr. Eduard G. Friedrich, Jr., who started the University of Florida Vulva Clinic. We acknowledge our colleagues, K Kendall Pierson, M.D., and Diane Mullins, M.D., who, as dermatopathologists, assisted with the diagnoses in a number of inflammatory and nevomelanocytic disorders. We acknowledge our colleagues in the International Society for the Study of Vulvar Disease, who have contributed significantly to our understanding of vulvar disease. We also acknowledge the secretarial assistance of Mrs. Sandra Fortier and Mrs. Debra Hope.

CONTENTS

CROSS-REFERENCE
TO
Histologic Classification of Vulvar Disease

GLOSSARY
AND
ADDITIONAL DISEASES OF THE VULVA

Acute Idiopathic Vulvar Ulcer: An acute, single, and painful ulcer of the medial aspect of the labia minora following within 24 hours of intercourse. The ulcer is of uncertain etiology.

Atopic Dermatitis: Inflammation associated with pruritus and burning of unknown etiology but may be mediated thorugh IgE and epidermal Langerhan's cells.

Contact Dermatitis: A cell-mediated inflammatory response secondary to a specific sensitizing agent, e.g., rubber, nickel, etc. Alternatively, an irritant-type inflammatory reaction secondary to exposure to a specific chemical or physical agent.

Facticial Vulvitis: Inflammation or ulceration of the vulva that is self-induced.

Fixed Drug Eruption (Dermatitis Medicamentosa): A urticarial, purpuric, bullous, maculopapular or other eruption of the vulva mediated by immunoglobulins (Types I and II), immunocomplexes (Type III), or cell mediated (Type IV) secondary to drug allergy.

Fox-Fordyce Disease: A disorder of apocrine glands associated with plugging of apocrine sweat ducts with keratin, causing severe pruritis and a papular eruption of the involved area.

Necrotizing Fasciitis (Synergistic Bacterial Infection): A life-threatening superficial and deep necrotizing inflammatory process of polymicrobial origin secondary to surgical trauma or injury.

Pyoderma Gangrenosum: A localized progressive ulcerative inflammatory process involving the vulvar skin, of unknown etiology.

Vulvitis Associated with Vaginitis: Inflammation of the vulva due to a specific vaginitis or vaginosis.

Vulvitis Granulomatosa: A granulomatous inflammatory process associated with edema, induration, and erythema of the labia majora and adjacent areas that may be associated with regional lymphadenoapthy.

Additional Cysts of the Vulva

Ciliated Cysts of the Vulvar Vestibule—Vestibular Adenosis: Cysts and surface epithelial changes characterized by tubal-endometrial-type epithelium. These changes in the vestibular epithelium, with squamous epithelium replaced by columnar epithelium, have been described secondary to acute inflammation of Stevens-Johnson syndrome, as well as secondary to 5-fluorouracil and/or laser therapy of the vestibule.

Cysts of the Canal of Nuck (Mesothelial Cysts): Simple cysts lined with peritoneum that are typically found in the superior labia majora or the inguinal canal.

Mesonephriclike Cyst (Wolfianlike Duct Cyst): Simple cysts of the vulva lined by cuboidal or columnar epithelium that is not ciliated and has smooth muscle beneath the epithelium.

Periurethral Cysts: Cysts found immediately adjacent to the urethra that may have a stratified squamous epithelial, transitional epithelial, or tall, pale mucos-secreting columnar epithelial lining.

Benign Epithelial Tumors

Ectopic Breast Tissue: Breastlike tissue within the vulva. Adenocarcinoma has been reported arising in vulvar breastlike tissue, as have other benign breast-type tumors.

Ectopic Salivary Gland Tissue: The finding of ectopic salivary gland within the vulva.

Keratoacanthoma: A benign but rapidly growing, self-limited epithelial neoplasm occurring on hair-bearing areas. The neoplasm has infiltrative margins and a keratin-filled crater. It regresses spontaneously if untreated.

Benign Vulvar Glandular Tumors

Adenoma of Minor Vestibular Glands: A benign, small (usually 1–2 mm) neoplasm composed of clustered mucin-secreting columnar epithelial-lined glands occurring within the vulvar vestibule; of minor vestibular gland origin.

Angiomyofibroblastoma: A benign tumor composed of spindled and oval stromal cells with relatively uniform, bland-appearing nuclei, eosinophilic cytoplasm, and infrequent or no mitosis. Numerous, variably shaped capillarylike vessels are present within the stromal component.

Dermatofibroma (Benign Fibrous Histiocytoma): The tumor is beneath the most superficial dermis and is composed of spindled fibroblast type-cells with a fascicular storiform growth pattern. The cell groups are separated in some areas by collagen.

Fibroma: A benign tumor of fibrous tissue origin composed of fibrocytes arranged in parallel and interlacing bundles.

Glomus Tumor: A benign tumor of smooth muscle or pericyte origin usually presenting as a painful solitary nodule less than 4 cm in diameter.

Leiomyoma: A benign tumor of smooth muscle origin composed of spindled interdigitated cells with relatively small, uniform nuclei without evident mitoses. Epitheloid leiomyoma has been decribed in the vulva.

Lipoma: A benign tumor arising from adipocytes composed of benign fat tissue with a supporting fibrovascular component.

Lymphangioma Circumscriptum: A benign disorder of localized dermal lymphatics characterized by the presentation of localized blebs and vesicles usually occurring in young women. Subepidermal multiloculated cystic lymphatic spaces, filled with acellular eosinophilic lymph, are found microscopically. The process is believed to be caused by a localized developmental defect of the superficial dermal lymphatics.

Mixed Tumor of the Vulva (Pleomorphic Adenoma): A benign tumor composed of epithelial tubules with a fibrous stromal element that may contain osseous, myxoid, and chondromatous components. The complex stromal component is believed to be of myoepithelial origin.

Neurofibroma: A benign tumor of nerve sheath origin that may be associated with Von Reclinghausen neurofibromatosis.

Nevus Lipomatous Superficialis: A congenital hamartoma of superficial connective tissue in which mature fat is present within the superficial dermis that is separate from the underlying subcutaneous fat.

Nodular Fasciitis (Aggressive Fibromatosus): A benign mass of myofibroblastic origin. Prominent vascularity, myoid change, and mitotic activity are common findings.

Nodular Hidradenoma (Clear-Cell Hidradenoma, Clear-Cell Myoblastoma, Clear-Cell Myoepithelioma, Solid Cystic Hidradenoma, Eccrine Acrospiroma, Eccrine Sweat Gland Tumor, Adenoma of Clear-Cell Type): A benign neoplasm of eccrine gland origin composed of glandular epithelial cells with distinctive clear cytoplasm.

Rhabdomyoma: A benign tumor of striated muscle origin composed of mature, well-differentiated rhabdomyoblasts.

Schwannoma (Neurilemoma): A tumor that arises from Schwann cells composed of densely packed spindle cells forming Antoni Type A areas admixed with hypocellular Antoni Type B areas. Benign and malignant variants of this tumor are described (see malignant Schwannoma).

Syringoma: A benign epithelial tumor arising from the ductal epithelium of the eccrine sweat gland characterized by small epithelial-lined ductlike structures that are round to comma shaped and form cysts containing eosinophilic secretion. The surrounding stroma or dermis is fibrous.

Trichilemmoma: A benign skin appendage tumor that contains amorphous keratin.

Trichoepithelioma: A benign tumor of hair follicle origin composed of small "horn cysts" containing keratin and surrounded by basaloid epithelial cells. Hair and/or hair-forming epithelial elements may be present.

Bullous Diseases

Benign Chronic Bullous Disease of Childhood (Linear IgA Disease): An acute bullous disorder usually associated with systemic symptoms, including fever and anorexia, that follows an acute bacterial or viral infection in approximately one-half of the cases. Lesions usually involve the genital and lower abdominal areas. The lesions become fully expressed within 1 day.

Bulla: A large circumscribed collection of fluid that may be between the epidermis and underlying dermis, or within the epidermis.

Darier's Disease: A congenital, multifocal acantholytic disorder inherited as an autosomal dominant trait.

Erythema Multiforme (Stevens-Johnson Syndrome): A systemic disorder that may follow infection, drug therapy, or radiotherapy, or following radiotherapy associated with keratinocyte hydropic degeneration and vesicle formation in the severe form (Stevens-Johnson syndrome). Intravascular deposition of complement and IgM can occur in the superficial vessels of the dermis.

Hailey-Hailey Disease (Familial Benign Pemphigus): A vesiculobullous disease that typically involves the intertriginous areas and is inherited as an autosomal dominant trait in nearly two-thirds of the cases.

Herpes Gestationis: An acute vesiculobullous eruption involving the skin of the genital area as well as abdomen and chest occurring exclusively in pregnant women, typically in the second trimester, related to complement fixing IgG antibodies.

Localized Acantholytic Disease of the Vulva: A papular inflammatory disorder that usually involves the labia majora and contigious skin of the medial thighs; of unknown etiology.

Vesicle: A small circumscribed collection of fluid within the skin.

Warty Dyskeratoma: A localized acantholytic disorder of unknown etiology.

Miscellaneous Disorders

Vulvar Amyloidosis: Involvement of the vulva with amyloidosis. Palpable vulvar nodules, formed by localized amyloid deposits, are the presenting feature.

Vulvar Calcinosis: Subcutaneous calcified nodules, typically 2 mm or less in diameter, associated with foreign body giant cells, mast cells, and chronic inflammation. The process is of unknown etiology.

Pigment Disorders

Acanthosis Nigricans and Pseudoacanthosis Nigricans: A velvety, brown-to-grey discoloration of vulvar skin, or skin of the axillac, inguinal folds or other sites. The involved skin is hyperkeratotic and has prominent acanthosis. The process may be related to one of three clinical situations: associated with visceral malignancies (acanthosis nigricans), found in obese patients (pseudoacanthosis), or found in children, unrelated to neoplasia or obesity.

Albinism: The absence of melanin, localized (piebaldism) or systemic, related to the inability of melanocytes to form melanin. This is an inherited disorder.

Congenital and Giant Nevomelanocytic Nevi: An inherited accumulation of nevomelanocytic cells. Congenital nevi are usually less than 4 cm in diameter, whereas giant nevomelanocytic nevi are 20 cm in diameter or larger.

Freckles (Ephelides): Localized excess melanin production. Freckles normally do not occur on the vulva.

Macule: A flat, nonelevated, discolored area on the skin.

Melanosis: Localized or multifocal macular pigmentation of the vulva that measures more than 4 mm in diameter.

Nevi—Junctional, Compound and Interdermal: Accumulations or nests of nevomelanocytic cells that are usually pigmented.

Papule: An elevated circumscribed area of the skin that is solid, not fluid-filled, and contiguous with the epithelium and/or superficial dermis. A papule may or may not be pigmented.

Postinflammatory Depigmentation (Leukoderma): The temporary absence or decrease of pigmentation and/or melanocytes due to trauma or ulceration.

Vitiligo: A localized loss of melanocytes and pigment within the skin. The disorder appears to be cell mediated in some cases and is recognized as an inherited disorder.

Reported Malignant Soft Tissue Tumors of the Vulva

Aggressive Angiomyxoma: A locally aggressive tumor composed of myxoid fibrous stroma with clustered small muscular arterioles of uncertain histogenesis.

Alveolar Soft-Part Sarcoma: This tumor forms rudimentary structures resembling pulmonary alveoli and is believed to be of striated muscle origin. This tumor has been reported as a primary tumor within the vulva.

Angiosarcoma: A malignant tumor of endothelial origin that forms endothelial-lined spaces that contain blood in the neoplastic vascular compartment. This tumor has been reported as a primary perianal tumor after radiation therapy to the pelvis.

Dermatofibrosarcoma Protuberans: A locally aggressive tumor of histiocytic origin that usually presents as a solitary, firm, brownish subcutaneous nodular or multinodular mass.

Embryonal Rhabdomyosarcoma (Sarcoma Botyroides): A malignant tumor of striated muscle origin that grows in a polypoid manner.

Epithelioid Sarcoma: A malignant soft tissue tumor with epithelial differentiation of uncertain histogenesis.

Granular Cell Tumor: A tumor of Schwann cell origin that has a distinctive granular cytoplasm. Although usually benign, locally aggressive and malignant granular cell tumors may occur in the vulva.

Langerhans Granulomatosis (Histiocytosis X), Including Eosinophilic Granuloma: A locally aggressive, or systemic, neoplasticlike histiocytic proliferation. Langerhans granulomatoses may present as one of three distinct clinical types. These include Letterer-Siwe disease, Hand-Schüller-Christian disease and eosinophilic granuloma. Of these, eosinophilic granuloma is by far the most common type involving the vulva.

Leiomyosarcoma: A malignant, smooth muscle tumor that usually arises from smooth muscle. It is the most common sarcoma of the vulva.

Liposarcoma: A malignant tumor arising from adipocytes and composed of neoplastic adipose tissue.

Lymphangiosarcoma: A malignant tumor of endothelial origin that forms endothelial-lined spaces that contain lymphatic fluid but do not contain blood.

Malignant Fibrous Histiocytoma: A malignant tumor that arises from histiocytes that have undergone fibroblastic differentiation. It is the second most common sarcoma of the vulva.

Malignant Rhabdoid Tumor: A malignant tumor of uncertain origin but which mimics striated muscle. This tumor has been reported presenting as a Bartholin mass in a young adult woman.

Malignant Schwannoma: A malignant tumor of Schwann cell origin. It has been reported arising within the labia minora and labia majora, as well as in other vulvar sites.

Primary Malignant Lymphoma: A malignant tumor of lymphocytic or hematopoietic stem cell origin. When arising in the vulva, this tumor can present as an ulcerative infiltrative lesion or as an expanding mass that can mimic a Bartholin gland neoplasm or clitoral enlargement. Kappa-positive lymphoplasmacytic lymphoma, angiocentric small and large mixed-cell lymphoma, and plasmocytoma have been reported arising in the vulva.

Yolk Sac Tumor (Endodermal Sinus Tumors): Primarily a germ cell tumor most commonly arising in the ovary or testis that is characterized by the formation of Schiller-Duval bodies and the production of α-fetoprotein. Its occurrence in extragonadal sites is rare. The vagina and vulva have been reported as primary sites.

1

INTRODUCTION

VULVAR ANATOMY

An understanding of the normal external anatomy of the vulva is of great value in recognizing pathologic changes, as well as guiding the pathologist to the appropriate differential should a biopsy be obtained. The epithelium of the vulva is highly variable, as are the type of subcutaneous tissues and accompanying skin appendages, if present. The key anatomic sites of the vulva are illustrated in Figure 1.1.

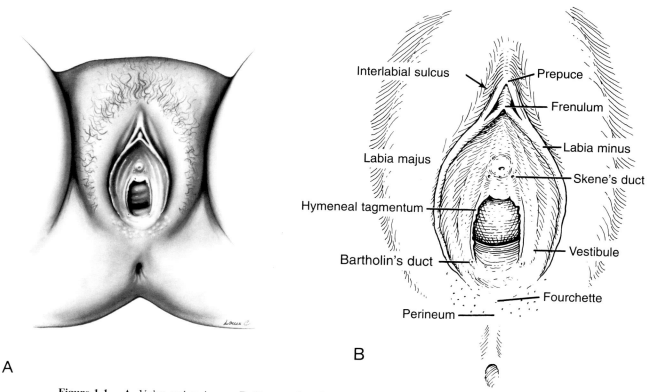

A

B

Interlabial sulcus

Prepuce

Frenulum

Labia minus

Skene's duct

Labia majus

Hymeneal tagmentum

Vestibule

Bartholin's duct

Fourchette

Perineum

Figure 1.1. **A.** Vulva and perineum. **B.** Topography of the vulva and perineum. (From Wilkinson EJ, Hardt NS. Vulva. In: Sternberg SS ed. Histology for pathologists. New York, Raven Press, 1992.)

VULVAR VESTIBULE

Definition

The portion of the vulva that extends from the exterior surface of the hymen to the frenulum of the clitoris anteriorly, fourchette posteriorly, and laterally to Hart's line where the nonkeratinized squamous epithelium of the vestibule joins the more papillated-appearing keratinized epithelium of the more lateral labia minora is the vulvar vestibule.

Epithelium

Stratified nonkeratinized squamous epithelium is approximately 1 mm thick (Figs. 1.2 and 1.3). Structures within the vulvar vestibule include:

1. urethral orifice,
2. openings of Skene's ducts,
3. vaginal introitus,
4. opening of Bartholin's ducts,
5. openings of the minor vestibular glands.

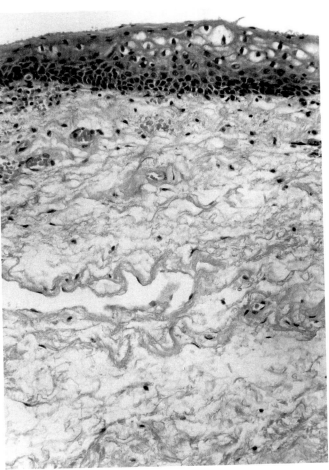

Figure 1.3. Vulvar vestibule, postmenopausal women. The epithelium is thin and nonkeratinized and has mild spongiosis. The subepithelial tissue contains many small vessels and is collagen rich.

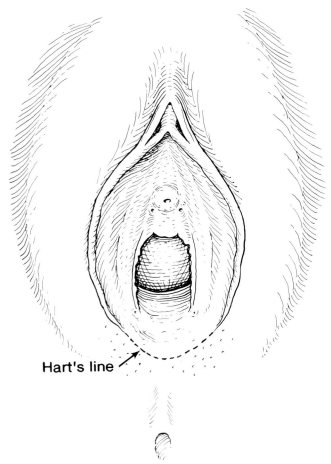

Hart's line

Figure 1.2. Hart's line defines the outer limits of the vulva vestibule. (From Wilkinson EJ, Hardt, NS. Vulva. In: Sternberg SS, ed. Histology for pathologists, New York, Raven Press, 1992.)

CLITORIS

The clitoris is homologous to the corpus cavernosum of the male penis. The clitoris consists of two crura and a glans clitoris. The crura are composed of erectile tissue that is enveloped by the tunica albuginea (Fig. 1.4). The clitoris has a length of 16 ± 1.4 mm, a transverse diameter of 3.4 ± 1.0 mm, and a longitudinal diameter of 5.1 ± 1.4 mm in adult women. Although height and weight do not influence size, parous women tend to have larger measurements.

Epithelium

The epithelium is squamous mucosa without glands, rete, or dermal papillae. The clitoris is rich in sensory receptors, as are the labia minora and majora.

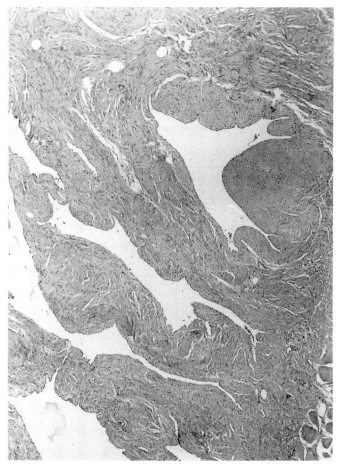

Figure 1.4. Erectile tissue. Prominent muscular vessels are vested by fibrous tissue. Striated muscle is seen in an adjacent area.

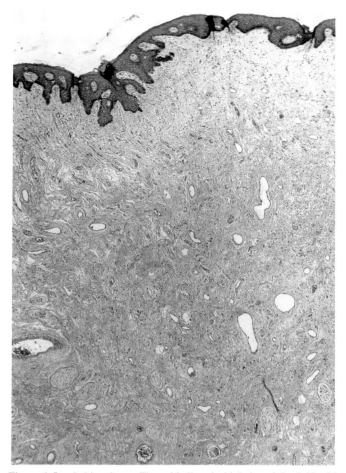

Figure 1.5. Labia minora. The epithelium is thinly keratinized. No skin appendages are present. The underlying dermis is highly vascular and collagen rich.

LABIA MINORA

The labia minora are separated laterally from the labia majora by the interlabial sulcus. The labia minora are homologous to the penile corpus spongiosis. The labia minora average approximately 5 cm in length and 0.5 cm in thickness, but length can vary considerably. Anteriorly the labia minora split, then fuse beneath the clitoris as the frenulum and above the clitoris to form the prepuce.

Epithelium

The epithelium of the labia minora is stratified squamous that is not keratinized on the vestibular surface and thinly keratinized on the lateral surface. In most women the labia minora do not contain skin appendages (Fig. 1.5).

Underlying Tissues

Although the labia minora are composed of erectile tissue supported by elastic tissue and are highly vascular, they lack adipose tissue. The ves-tibular bulbs are deep to the labia minora and are composed of erectile tissue supported by the bulbocavernosus muscles.

LABIA MAJORA

Medially the labia majora are bounded by the intralabial sulcus, the labia minora, and the vulvar vestibule. Laterally the labia majora are bounded by, and merge with, the inguinal-gluteal folds, which separate the labia majora from the thighs. The increase in size of the labia majora with puberty is predominantly associated with an increase in subcutaneous fat of the labia majora. Anteriorly the labia majora fuse with the mons pubis, and with the perineal body posteriorly.

Epithelium

The labia majora are covered with stratified squamous epithelium, which is hair-bearing in the lateral and midportions of the labial surface, and hairless in its medial surfaces. These hair shafts are associated with sebaceous glands and apocrine sweat glands in pilosebaceous units (Fig. 1.6). Medially sebaceous glands enter the epithelium directly, independent of hair (Fig. 1.7). These sebaceous glands on the medial aspects of the labia majora can be seen clinically as Fordyce spots. At the inferior medial aspects of the labia majora, the sebaceous gland elements are lost medial to Hart's line, which marks the lateral posterior boundary of the vestibule.

Both sebaceous and apocrine glands are stimulated by sex hormones; however, the merocrine sweat glands are functional throughout life. The sebaceous glands of the labia majora measure up to 2.03 mm in depth. Hair follicles measure up to 2.38 mm in depth. Within the mons pubis the hair follicle depth may be up to 2.72 mm. The normal epithelium of non-hair-bearing or non-gland-bearing regions of the vulva is approximately 1 mm thick.

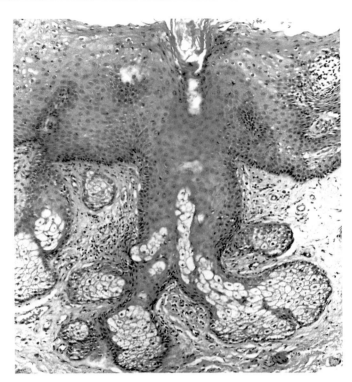

Figure 1.7. Labia majora, medial aspect. Sebaceous glands open directly to the surface.

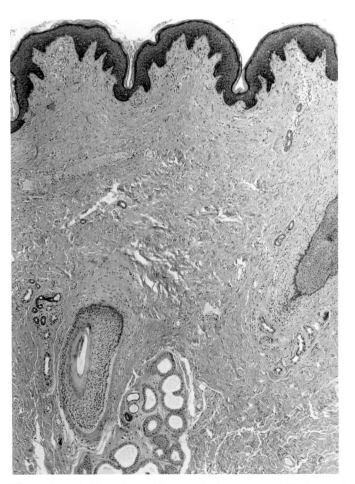

Figure 1.6. Labia majora with keratinized squamous epithelium and associated hair follicle and apocrine glands.

Underlying Tissues

Within the anterior labia majora, adjacent and external to the inguinal canal, a deep smooth muscle layer (cremaster muscle) is found that joins superiorly with the round ligament. Entrapped peritoneum (processus vaginalis) within the round ligament may result in a cyst of the canal of Nuck, resulting in labial enlargement. These cysts may mimic inguinal hernia.

The collagen-rich dermis of the vulva contains many fibroblasts that, in pregnancy, have myofibroblastic differentiation. The contractile ability of these myofibroblasts is believed to be involved in the rapid return of the vulva and vagina to normal within the postpartum period (Wilkinson, 1991).

MONS PUBIS

The mons is that portion of the vulva presenting as the rounded, fleshy prominence over the symphysis pubis. The mons epithelium is composed of stratified squamous epithelium, which is hair bearing. The skin of the mons is similar to that of the labia majora with pilosebaceous units distributed throughout its substance. Hair follicle depth may be up to 2.72 mm. The underlying tissue of the mons is composed primarily of adipose tissue.

GENERAL FEATURES

Vulvar pathology will account for fewer than 5% of new gynecologic patient visits. The majority of vulvar complaints will involve conditions that will require long-term management and that, in many instances, will be incurable. A busy vulvar clinic may find 40% of its new patients complaining of dyspareunia secondary to symptoms of vestibulitis (Fig. 1.8). Fourteen percent of patients may have human papillomavirus-associated conditions such as condylomata and vulvar intraepithelial neoplasia. Thirteen percent of patients may complain of the chronic pruritus of lichen sclerosus. Nonspecific vulvitis may account for 7% of new patient visits. Lichen planus may be seen in 5% of patients. Essential vulvodynia may account for 5% of new visits. These six diagnoses may account for approximately 83% of new visits to a vulva clinic. They will also account for the majority of the return visits because they will require long-term management decisions.

The remaining vulvar pathology will comprise various dermatologic conditions, which may be infectious, inflammatory, or neoplastic.

CLINICAL PRESENTATION

The most common patient complaint resulting in evaluation in a vulva clinic will be pain, such as noted with vestibulitis, lichen planus, and essential vulvodynia. The second most frequent symptom will be pruritus, observed especially in lichen sclerosus and nonspecific vulvitis. Patients may also present with complaints of palpable masses on the vulva (human papillomavirus-associated conditions, such as vulvar intraepithelial neoplasia and condyloma acuminatum). A detailed history will assist in defining symptoms and contributing factors (Fig. 1.9).

Classification will be based upon the visual clinical presentation of vulvar disease. Lesions will be distinguished primarily by their surface contour. A macule is a flat lesion, demonstrating no elevation above contiguous skin. A papule is a well-defined, elevated lesion with solid matrix. A plaque is an elevated relatively flat area of skin. A verruca is an elevated lesion with a horny appearance. An erosion is a defect resulting from partial loss of the epithelium. An ulcer is a depressed defect in the normal skin that results from destruction or loss of the dermis and epidermis. A tumor is a neoplasm within the skin or the subcuticular tissue. When the

basic architecture of the vulvar lesion has been defined, lesions may be characterized further by their color. Often these two parameters, architecture and color, alone will suffice for assigning a diagnosis and initiating therapy.

Magnified imaging of the vulva with the colposcope is useful when examining melanotic lesions for border regularity. More frequently the colposcope is used to define the extent of vulvar intraepithelial neoplasia. The evaluation is particularly productive when the patient has held a gauze saturated with 3% to 5% acetic acid (or white vinegar) against the vulva for several minutes before colposcopic magnification. A green filter will enhance definition of the multifocal lesions.

Certain entities require histologic diagnosis to initiate therapy and to rule out malignancy. The usefulness of histology is of special note in the evaluation of hyperpigmented lesions. It is difficult clinically to discern the diagnosis of melanotic lesions. They may range in significance from the insignificant lentigo simplex to the more ominous dysplastic nevus and the potentially fatal melanoma. Only the pathologist can define the diagnosis after reviewing a representative biopsy performed by the clinician.

Biopsies of vulvar tissue should be performed under sterile conditions and after appropriate preparation of the skin with an antiseptic solution. Local infiltration with 1% lidocaine provides adequate anesthesia. Occasionally, tender, inflamed lesions may benefit from a topical preanesthetic 20% benzocaine spray (Hurricaine) before infiltration with lidocaine. Although the Keyes punch biopsy may be used to sample vulvar lesions, the no. 15 blade scalpel will allow a much larger representative specimen to be removed and often will allow complete excisional biopsy for histologic evaluation. The depth of incision can be controlled more easily when using the scalpel than when using the Keyes punch biopsy. Vulvar hematomas have resulted from use of a sharp Keyes punch biopsy pressed too deeply into the subcuticular tissue. Closure of the biopsy site is easily accomplished with chromic gut. Although delayed absorbable suture material such as polyglactin 910 may be used, the knots on these materials often become a nuisance and patients return requesting removal. The skin of the vulva is relatively lax and rarely requires undermining for the closure of excisions. Excisional biopsies performed in tissue planes, which are under tension at closure or which are at risk of delayed healing, may

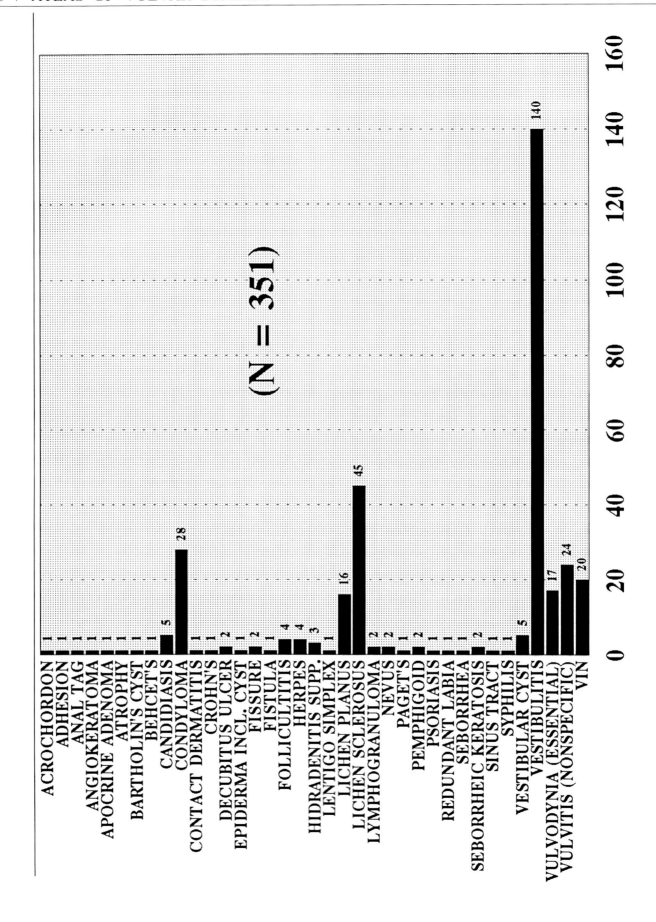

Patient Name: _____ MR #: _____

Vulvovaginal Consultation

Name: _____ Date: _____ Age: _____

Ht.: _____ Wt.: _____ Race: ☐ White ☐ Black ☐ Asian ☐ Hisp. ☐ Other _____

Marital Status: ☐ Married ☐ Single ☐ Widowed ☐ Divorced Parity:

Term	Prem	AB	Living

LMP: _____ Contraception: _____

Menstrual Hygiene: ☐ N/A ☐ Tampons ☐ Pads ☐ Both ☐ Deodorant Coital Frequency: _____

Occupation: _____ Sports/Exercise: _____

Present Illness: _____

Major Symptoms: _____

_____ Duration: _____

Changed by: ☐ Coitus ☐ Menses ☐ Clothing ☐ Position/Activity ☐ Diet ☐ Other _____

Similar Disease in Family/Partner: _____ On Other Body Sites: _____

Recent Therapy: _____

Relevant History: _____

Surgical: _____ Psychiatric: _____

Medical: _____ Medication: _____

Foreign Travel: _____

Spinal Injury, Surgery, or Symptoms: _____

Estrogen Replacement: _____ Allergies: _____ Diabetes: Family _____ Self _____

Prior Vaginitis: _____ HPV: _____ HSV: _____ Other STD: _____

Underwear Fabric: _____ Laundry Products Now Used: _____ Incontinence: _____

Vulvar Hygiene: _____ Douche Hx.: _____

Hot Tub/Spa: _____ Ever Catheterized? _____

Description of Findings: _____

Vulva: _____

Attach Photo

Sketch Lesion
Indicate Biopsy Site ⊗

Vagina: Cells: ☐ Clue ☐ WBC

pH: _____ Flora: _____

Discharge: _____

Mucosa: _____

Cervix: _____

Bimanual: _____

Initial Impression: _____

_____

_____

Plan: _____

_____

_____

_____

_____ , MD
Director/Attending

require placement of permanent suture material for 10 days to effect apposition. Small-gauge (5-0) monofilament nylon may be placed in an interrupted mattress stitch.

Care should be taken when considering excising large melanotic lesions. If the clinical suspicion of a large lesion is melanoma, then a representative biopsy of the thickest region of the melanoma should be obtained. If the diagnosis of melanoma is confirmed and the patient is a candidate for excision, this should be accomplished in the operating room. There, more appropriate margins may be obtained to confirm containment of the melanoma within the histologic specimen. Similarly, a patient with Paget's disease may have a representative biopsy taken in the clinic but should be treated with therapeutic excision in the operating room to confirm removal of all involved tissue.

Occasionally tissue should also be sent for immunohistology. This may be extremely helpful in evaluating a patient with a presumed diagnosis of pemphigus. Tissue removed for routine histology may be split and one portion placed in Michel's solution for direct immunohistology.

ADJUNCTIVE STUDIES

Adjunctive studies are of particular importance in evaluating patients who present with ulcers. It is difficult to discern, purely on clinical grounds, the etiology of vulvar ulceration. The differential includes conditions which require further laboratory evaluation to include herpes cultures, dark-field microscopy for *Treponema,* serologic studies for syphilis (venereal disease rise or RPR), serologic studies for human immunodeficiency virus, serology for lymphogranuloma venereum (*Chlamydia*), and cultures for *Haemophilus ducreyi.* Certain ulcerative conditions will require histologic evaluation to rule out carcinoma or the vasculitis of Behçet's syndrome.

Cervical cytology should be obtained on patients as a matter of routine, but especially in patients who have evidence of vulvar intraepithelial neoplasia. This multifocal disease often involves the cervix and vulva concomitantly. The same is true for condyloma acuminatum. The patient with vulvar condylomata will frequently have vaginal and cervical disease and any therapeutic approach should include the appropriate clinical evaluation of the vagina and cervix before treatment is started.

Bimanual examination should be included in the evaluation as a matter of routine. Many of the conditions that affect the vulva occur in older women, and rectovaginal examination may demonstrate pathology that may be contributing to the vulvar condition or that may be a separate clinical concern, such as colonic carcinoma.

For certain conditions of the vulva, an extensive evaluation to rule out carcinoma in other extragenital sites is necessary. The primary condition mandating such an evaluation is Paget's disease. Appropriate evaluation of the breasts, colon, and urologic system should be concluded before treatment.

DIFFERENTIAL DIAGNOSIS

Many vulvar conditions (and skin conditions in general) may be confused with one another on clinical grounds. Even after a complete histologic and adjunctive evaluation, diagnostic uncertainty may remain. In certain conditions this may be moot, if there is no possibility of malignancy and the conditions are treated identically, regardless of diagnosis (i.e., the pruritus of lichen simplex chronicus and the pruritus of seborrhea are both managed with topical steroids).

CLINICAL BEHAVIOR AND TREATMENT

Many vulvar conditions are recalcitrant and difficult to manage. They will require frequent and long-term communication between the patient and the physician. The patient must understand that many dermatologic conditions cannot be cured and that the ultimate goal is containment of symptoms leading to improved quality of life. Sometimes, this will require what the patient may view as inappropriate therapy (i.e., tricyclic antidepressant therapy for essential vulvodynia). An understanding physician may spend numerous sessions allaying the patient's anxiety and explaining to the spouse why an antidepressant is being prescribed for pain.

Pruritic vulvar conditions are usually easily treated. If the primary condition is infectious and due to *Candida,* the underlying pathology may be corrected easily. This is not so for patients who suffer from the pruritus of lichen sclerosus. The underlying pathology is a permanent condition and cannot be cured; however, the pruritus is easily managed with topical steroid therapy. Pruritus may also be relieved on occasion with oral antihistamine preparations such as hydroxyzine (Atarax), but such preparations lack antiinflammatory properties and have no direct effect on the primary condition.

Another condition associated with long-term potential for recurrence is infection with human papillomavirus (condylomata acuminata and vulvar intraepithelial neoplasia). The patient will require extensive counseling concerning the necessity for long-term follow-up. She must understand that after therapy she may reacquire the virus or it may persist in normal skin, recurring later. Repeated laser ablations may be necessary and pharmacologic augmentation with 5% 5-fluorouracil and/or interferon may be required to control the disease. The clinician should never assure the patient that human papilloma virus has been eradicated from the vulva. Such an assurance will too frequently lead to professional embarrassment when the disease recurs several weeks to several months after expensive therapy.

Progressive Therapeutic Options

Often there are a number of options available to the clinician managing vulvar disease. In rare instances, lesions may be observed without therapeutic intervention. The classic keratinous cyst noted in the pilosebaceous area of the vulva requires no management unless associated with symptoms. Other lesions of the vulva require excision immediately upon observation. Solid tumors and melanotic lesions of the vulva should be removed to rule out malignancy.

Other conditions such as condylomata acuminata may have a range of therapeutic options beginning with less invasive and more economical options. Focal disease may be managed in the clinic with inexpensive topical desiccants; however, diffuse disease will require expensive laser ablation and use of topical 5%-fluorouracil or injectable interferons.

Therapeutic approaches should be tailored to the extent of the disease and the patient's ability to adhere to therapeutic recommendations. Side effects should be minimized. Recommendations should be fiscally sound. If the first option fails, then progress through the remaining options until *(a)* the disease is cured or controlled, *(b)* adverse side effects are encountered, *(c)* the expense becomes prohibitive, or *(d)* lack of experience precludes use (i.e., immunosuppressants, laser therapy, etc.).

SUGGESTED READING LIST

Dickinson RL. Human sex anatomy. 2nd ed. Baltimore: Williams & Wilkins, 1949.
Edwards JNT, Morris HB. Langerhans cells and lymphocyte subsets in the female genital tract. Br J Obstet Gynaecol 1985;92:974–982.
Fetissof F, Berger G, Dubois MP, et al. Endocrine cells in the female genital tract. Histopathology 1985;9:133–145.
Friedrich EG, Jr. Vulvar disease. Philadelphia: WB Saunders, 1983.
Friedrich EG, Jr. Vulvar vestibulitis syndrome. J Reprod Med 1987;32:110–114.
Friedrich EG, Jr, Wilkinson EJ. Mucous cysts of the vulvar vestibule. Obstet Gynecol 1973;42:407–414.
Growdon WA, Fu Y, Lebberz TB, Rapkin A, Mason GD, Parks G. Pruritic vulvar squamous papillomatosis: evidence for human papillomavirus etiology. Obstet Gynecol 1985;66:564–568.
Hu F. Melanocyte cytology in normal skin. In: Ackerman AB, ed. Masson Monographs in Dermatology-1. New York: Masson, 1981.
Kaufman RH, Friedrich EG, Gardner HL. Benign diseases of the vulva and vagina. 3rd ed. Chicago: Year Book Medical Publishers, 1989.
Krantz KE. Innervation of the human vulva and vagina. Obstet Gynecol 1958;12:382–396.
Krantz KE. The anatomy and physiology of the vulva and vagina. In: Philipp EE, Barnes J, Newton M, eds. Scientific foundation of obstetrics and gynaecology. 2nd ed. London: Heinemann, 1977:65–78.
Lunde O. A study of body hair density and distribution in normal women. Am J Phys Anthropol 1984;64:179–184.
McKay M. Subsets of vulvodynia. J Reprod Med 1988;33:695–698.
Parmley T. Embryology of the female genital tract. In: Kurman RJ, ed. Blaustein's pathology of the female genital tract, 3rd ed. New York: Springer Verlag, 1987:1–14.
Pyka R, Wilkinson EJ, Friedrich EG, Croker BP. The histology of vulvar vestibulitis syndrome. Int J Gynecol Oncol 1988;7:249–257.
Reid R, Greenberg MD, Daoud Y, Selvaggi S, Husain M, Wilkinson EJ: Colposcopic findings in women with vulvar pain syndromes: a preliminary report. J Reprod Med 1988;33:523–532.
Ridley CM. The vulva. New York: Churchill Livingstone, 1988:1–69.
Robboy SJ, Ross JS, Prat J, Keh PC, Welch WR. Urogenital sinus origin of mucinous and ciliated cysts of the vulva. Obstet Gynecol 1978;51:347–351.
Rorat E, Ferenczy A, Richart RM. Human Bartholin gland, duct, and duct cyst. Arch Pathol 1975;99:367–374.
Shatz P, Bergeron C, Wilkinson EJ, Arseneau J, Ferenczy A. Vulvar intraepithelial neoplasia and skin appendage involvement. Obstet Gynecol 1989;74:769–774.
Verkauf BS, Von Thron J, O'Brien WF. Clitoral size in normal women. Obstet Gynecol 1992;80:41–44.
Wilkinson EJ. Pathology of the vagina. Curr Opin Obstet Gynecol 1991;3:553.
Wilkinson EJ, Friedrich EG, Jr. Diseases of the vulva. In: Kurman RJ, ed. Blaustein's pathology of the female genital tract. 3rd ed. New York: Springer Verlag, 1987:36–96.
Wilkinson EJ, Hardt NS. Histology of the vulva. In: Sternberg SS, ed. Histology for pathologists. New York: Raven Press, 1991.
Word B. Office treatment of cyst and abscess of Bartholin's gland duct. South Med J 1968;61:514–518.

2

CYSTS

CYST ALGORITHM

CYST (Greek kystis: sac, bladder): cavity, lined by epithelium, containing a liquid or semisolid material.

Location	Presumed Diagnosis
Vestibule	Bartholin's cyst/abscess
	Mucous cyst
	Skene's duct cyst
Labium minus	Mucous cyst
Labium majus	Epidermal inclusion cyst

Figure 2.1. Cyst algorithm.

Bartholin's Cyst/Abscess

DEFINITION

Obstruction of the ductal system of the Bartholin's gland results in formation of one or more cysts. An obstructed, infected gland may form an abscess.

GENERAL FEATURES

Cyst and abscess formation of the Bartholin's gland will account for the majority of symptomatic vulvar cysts observed in a gynecology practice.

CLINICAL PRESENTATION

A Bartholin's cyst may create a pressure phenomenon at the introitus. The usual asymptomatic cyst is 1–2 cm in diameter; however, cysts often are much larger. The usual location is at the posterior introitus in the region of the duct opening into the vestibule. Larger cysts will protrude medially, obscuring the normal introital opening. Occasionally cysts will dissect anteriorly within the body of the labium majus and laterally into the subcutaneous fat lateral to the introitus. The most severely symptomatic patient will present with evidence of an infection in the Bartholin's gland. This infection will have progressed to abscess formation. It is by no means a prerequisite that a Bartholin's cyst be present before an abscess develops. Acute obstruction of the Bartholin's duct secondary to infection may eventuate in rapid development of an abscess over 2–5 days. Based upon the severity of the infection, and the infecting organism, the patient may appear septic. Although *Neisseria gonorrhoeae* historically has been associated with Bartholin's gland abscess formation, other organisms are more frequently isolated, especially anaerobes. Organisms that produce exotoxins may lead to toxic shock.

The diagnosis of a Bartholin's cyst is readily made on physical examination. The classic, medially protruding cystic structure at the posterior introitus is almost invariably a Bartholin's cyst. Minor vestibular cysts are much smaller and are quite superficial at the introital opening, just inferior to the hymen. The Bartholin's cyst is much more deeply seated and typically larger. Lipomas may present at the introitus, but are usually observed in the labium majus and are often lobulated or shaped like a sausage. Abscess formation in the Bartholin's gland is suspected when the classically located mass is tender. Often the well-developed abscess will have an attenuated epithelial lining at the introitus, a sign of a pointing abscess. There will be induration around the gland. The abscess may dissect into the labium majus, especially if the abscess is multilocular.

Of special concern in a patient with a Bartholin's process is the potential for the development of carcinoma. The classic presentation is that of an irregular, nodular mass in the region of the Bartholin's gland in a postmenopausal woman. Younger women have been noted to develop carcinoma of the Bartholin's gland and this diagnosis should be considered in all patients with nodularity, irregularity, or persistent induration.

MICROSCOPIC FINDINGS

The Bartholin's cyst arises primarily from obstruction of the distal Bartholin's duct. The secretion within the dilated duct is clear, mucoid, translucent, bacteria free, and essentially acellular. This represents secretion of sialomucin from the Bartholin's glands. The secretion stains with mucin and periodic acid-Schiff stain, both before and after diastase digestion and Alcian blue at pH 2.5. These are the same staining features found in the cytoplasm of the secretory epithelium of the Bartholin's gland.

Bartholin's cysts are lined with Bartholin's duct-type epithelium, which is usually flattened transitional or squamous-type epithelium. The cyst epithelium is typically found adjacent to normal Bartholin's glandular epithelium. The adjacent stroma is usually normal and inflammation may be seen in the adjacent stroma. In some cases, mucocelelike changes may be seen, where secretion is found within the stroma, having dissected into the stroma from rupture and leakage of the cyst. Foamy histiocytes may also be seen in the stroma. In such cases, the adjacent Bartholin's gland tissues are nodular and contain small cysts.

CLINICAL BEHAVIOR AND TREATMENT

The asymptomatic smooth Bartholin's cyst requires no intervention. Symptomatic cysts and abscesses will require drainage. The most efficacious and readily performed procedure is drainage of the cyst or abscess by placement of a Word catheter. The Word catheter contains a small inflatable balloon into which 2–3 mL of solution may be injected to allow retention of the catheter within the cavity of the Bartholin's cyst or abscess. If the cyst is smaller than the balloon, it will not be feasible to use the catheter. The cyst or abscess should be readily attainable, or pointing at the introitus. It is extremely difficult to place a Word catheter within a deep-seated Bartholin's cyst or abscess, especially one of small size. After obtaining local anesthesia over the region of the normal gland opening at the introitus, a no. 11 blade is used to make a stab incision into the Bartholin's cavity. This incision should not be excessively wide because the balloon must be retained within the cavity. If the contents of the cavity appear to be infected, appropriate cultures should be obtained for pathogens, especially *N. gonorrhoeae*. It is not cost-effective to obtain cultures for anaerobes. If there is evidence of periglandular induration and inflammation, consideration should be given to initiating oral antibiotic therapy with a broad-spectrum antibiotic. Signs of sepsis should prompt intravenous therapy with coverage for coagulase-positive staphylococcal organisms. Until cultures have returned, antibiotic coverage should also be directed against *N. gonorrhoeae*. If an abscess is suspected, but is not fully formed and is not pointing, the patient should be managed with hot soaks or sitz baths and oral antibiotics until the abscess cavity is fluctuant and identifiable. It is not necessary to hospitalize the patient for this therapy unless she is unable to take oral antibiotics or appears obviously septic. It is important to emphasize that the incision used to drain a cyst or abscess should be placed just inferior (exterior) to the hymenal ring within the introitus in the region of the normal gland opening. It is not appropriate to place this incision on the external genitalia. The placement of an incision on the external genitalia may rarely be necessary when an abscess is pointing in this region and rupture is imminent.

An alternative to drainage of a Bartholin's cyst with a Word catheter is marsupialization of the cyst. This may be accomplished in the office with appropriate anesthesia; however, frequently, more substantial anesthesia is necessary and performance in the operating room may be more appropriate. The vestibular skin overlying the Bartholin's cyst is incised in a cruciate fashion. The cyst is entered and drained of its contents. An effort is made to determine that the cyst is unilocular. The apices of the cruciate skin incision are excised and the epithelium of the cyst is sutured to the edge of the vestibular skin in an interrupted fashion. This creates an orifice that will heal and allow continued drainage of the Bartholin's cyst. An alternative approach is laser creation of a tract into the Bartholin's cyst; however, this is not a universally available nor frequently attempted approach. Marsupialization of an infected gland should not be attempted. The Word catheter placement is the preferred management for an abscess. The catheter should be left in place for 4–6 weeks to permit epithelialization of a tract. Patients with findings suggestive of the possibility of carcinoma should have excisional biopsies performed. The mass should be removed and submitted for pathologic examination. If pathology demonstrates carcinoma, more radical surgery will be necessary for definitive therapy and to define the extent of disease.

Rarely, it will be necessary to excise a deeply seated Bartholin's cyst that is symptomatic and not readily approachable with a Word catheter. The vascularity in the periglandular region may be significant, especially if there has been long-standing inflammation. Dissection will be tedious and meticulous hemostasis will be necessary. Postoperative hematoma formation and/or infection may result. Chronic scarring, perhaps present before surgery, and certainly a possibility after surgery, may lead to long-term dyspareunia. The patient should be advised of these possibilities.

Progressive Therapeutic Options

1. Observe without intervention the asymptomatic, smooth Bartholin's cyst.

2. Insert a Word catheter under appropriate local anesthesia for the symptomatic Bartholin's cyst or for the Bartholin's abscess pointing at the introitus. Allow the catheter to remain in situ for 4–6 weeks to allow epithelization of the Bartholin's tract. The Word catheter should be inserted in the posterior aspect of the introitus just inferior (exterior) to the hymenal ring in the normal location of the Bartholin's duct opening.

3. Marsupialize symptomatic cysts if a Word catheter is not available or if a Word catheter has previously failed to maintain an epithelial tract.

4. Excise Bartholin's cysts that are symptomatic and have failed to respond to Word catheter placement or marsupialization.

5. Excise all persistently irregular masses in the region of the Bartholin's gland, especially in perimenopausal and postmenopausal women, to rule out carcinoma.

NOTATION: Culture all Bartholin's abscesses for *N. gonorrhoeae*.

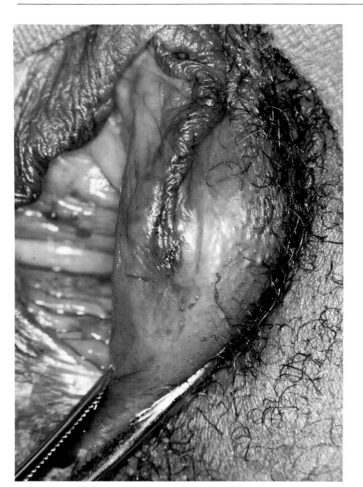

Figure 2.2. Persistent Bartholin's gland with induration that required excision in the operating room. Histologic study revealed that the cyst was benign.

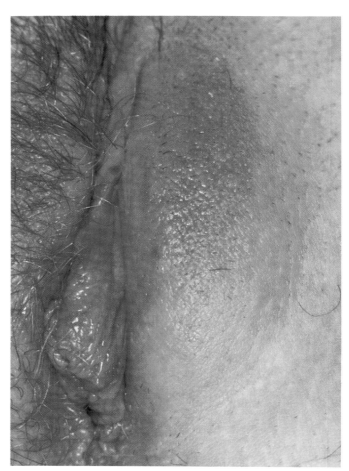

Figure 2.3. Bartholin's cyst dissecting anteriorly to the border of the left labium majus, originally thought to be a canal of Nuck cyst.

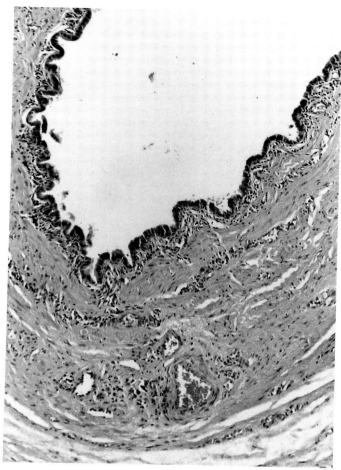

Figure 2.4. Bartholin's duct cyst. A slightly flattened columnar epithelium is seen lining this cyst.

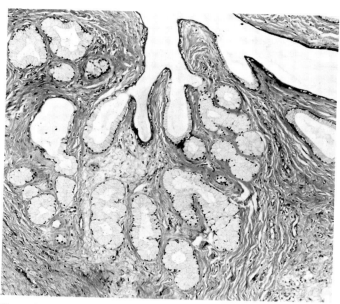

Figure 2.5. Bartholin's gland and contiguous dilated duct. The dilated duct contains inspissated mucoid secretion. The glands are lined by a tall, mucus-secreting columnar epithelium. The transitional area from the secretory to the ductal epithelium is evident.

Keratinous Cyst (Epidermial Inclusion Cyst)

DEFINITION

An epidermal inclusion cyst is a cystic structure lined with stratified squamous epithelium.

GENERAL FEATURES

The etiology is obscure but may be secondary to trauma, with subsequent entrapment of epidermis within dermal tissue. Alternatively epidermal inclusion cysts may be a consequence of developmental entrapment of epidermis within dermis or may be a consequence of obstruction of pilosebaceous ducts and glands.

CLINICAL PRESENTATION

Most commonly, patients with epidermal inclusion cysts will present complaining of palpable nodularity within the skin of the vulva. On rare occasions a patient may present with an infected inclusion cyst and complain of marked tenderness in the region. Typically the uninfected epidermal inclusion cyst is asymptomatic. An exceedingly rare complication is the development of squamous cell carcinoma within the cyst.

Examination of the vulva may demonstrate multiple nodules within the skin of the labia majora. These will be mobile and nontender. Often they will be contiguous. Close examination will reveal a small opening on the surface of the nodule that may be plugged with keratin. Pressure will often result in extravasation of the keratin plug and the keratin content of the inclusion cyst.

The diagnosis of an epidermal inclusion cyst is easily made by observation. Confirmation of diagnosis may be obtained by excision of the cyst and submission for pathologic studies.

MICROSCOPIC FINDINGS

Excised vulvar keratinous cysts typically range from 2 to 5 mm in diameter and are superficial. These cysts contain a white to yellow grumous material. The lining is typically a nonkeratinized squamous epithelium without a granular layer. Other types of skin appendage cysts may also be seen within the vulva that should be distinguished from keratinous cysts.

Within the dermal tissues adjacent to the cyst, foreign body-type giant cells may be seen with associated chronic inflammation. In these cases, the keratinous material may be found in the adjacent tissue secondary to rupture and leakage of the contents of the cyst into the dermis.

CLINICAL BEHAVIOR AND TREATMENT

Usually epidermal inclusion cysts require no therapy. The patient may be reassured that these cysts are benign and that malignant changes have been extremely rare. If after discussing this issue with the patient, she desires removal, this may be accomplished easily in the clinic setting. Drainage of the cyst will not be therapeutic. The stratified squamous epithelium will continue to desquamate within the cystic wall and the cyst will recur. The cyst must be excised. Solitary cysts or multiple contiguous cysts may be excised easily after accomplishing local anesthesia with lidocaine. The skin overlying the cyst or cysts is incised and a small hemostat will be helpful in grasping the cyst wall and extracting it from the dermis. Solitary small lesions will require no suture placement; however, multiple contiguous cysts requiring a lengthy incision or a large solitary cyst requiring a large incision will require placement of sutures for skin apposition.

An infected epidermal inclusion cyst will require hot soaks to enhance loculation and oral antibiotics to control the infection. Antibiotics should be continued until the local erythema and induration have subsided. Drainage should be accomplished if an abscess forms. The inclusion cyst may be removed after the infection has completely resolved and no induration or erythema persists.

Progressive Therapeutic Options

1. Reassure the patient that the epidermal inclusion cyst is rarely a problem and may be followed without removal.
2. Based upon the patient's desires, or symptoms, excision of the cyst may be accomplished under local anesthesia.
3. The presence of inflammation requires antibiotic therapy and precludes excision until the inflammation has subsided.

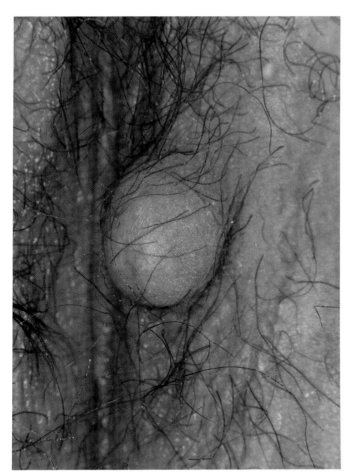

Figure 2.6. Epidermal inclusion cyst excised in clinic.

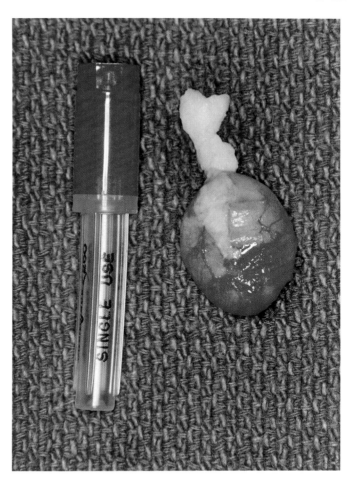

Figure 2.7. Excised epidermal inclusion cyst. Note the sebaceous-appearing material.

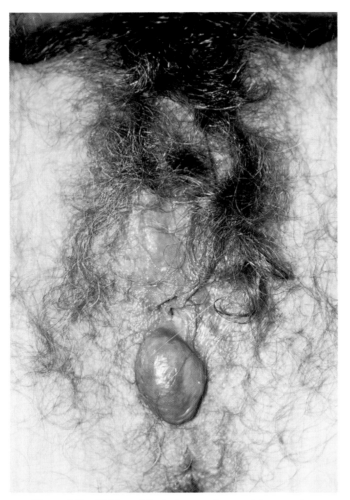

Figure 2.8. Epidermal inclusion cyst in an episiotomy site.

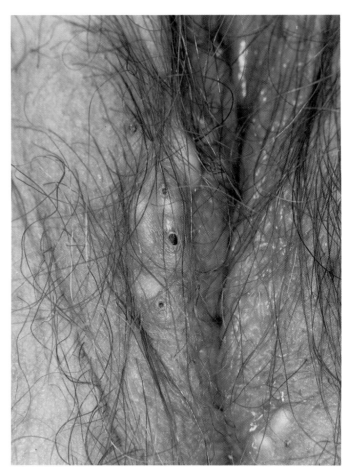

Figure 2.9. Multiple epidermal inclusion cysts with keratin plugs.

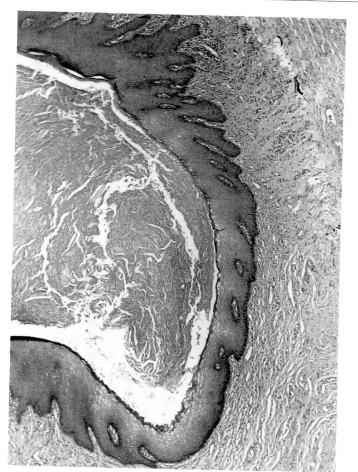

Figure 2.10. Epidermal inclusion cyst. Exfoliated squamous epithelial cells are present within the cyst lumen. The lining is stratified squamous epithelium. Fibrovascular tissue surrounds this cyst and is within normal limits.

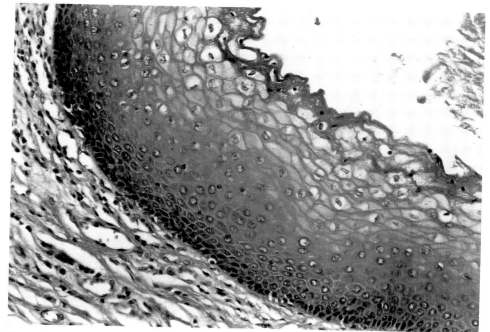

Figure 2.11. Higher magnification of the adjacent field demonstrates the nonkeratinized stratified squamous epithelial lining.

Skene's Duct Cyst

DEFINITION

Skene's duct cysts are cystic dilations of the Skene's glands usually located adjacent to the urethral meatus within the vulvar vestibule.

GENERAL FEATURES

Periurethral cysts may be found along the entire length of the posterior and lateral urethra; however, those cysts involving the distal urethra are usually visible as periurethral cysts within the vestibule. Their origin may be a consequence of congenital hypoplasia of the Skene's duct or acquired stricture or obstruction of the duct, usually as a consequence of inflammation.

CLINICAL PRESENTATION

The orifices of Skene's ducts are usually visible as bilateral single small opening adjacent to the urethral meatus (see Fig. 1.1B). Although Skene's duct cysts are relatively uncommon, when they are observed it is usually during a routine vaginal examination, although an occasional patient may have specific complaints, usually referable to dysuria or changes in the urinary stream. Because most Skene's duct cysts are small, they rarely interfere with urination; however, a large, dilated Skene's cyst may result in urinary diversion and a complaint of lateral spraying of urine. With continued dilatation of the cyst, urinary obstruction may be a consequence.

The diagnosis is suspected upon visualizing a vestibular cyst that is inferior or lateral to the urethral meatus (Fig. 2.12). Slight tenderness may be observed with compression, although the cysts are usually not tender. A tender periurethral mass suggests secondary infection, which is a rare complication of Skene's duct cysts. The asymptomatic cyst will require no further evaluation. The patient with symptoms will warrant further consideration before therapy.

MICROSCOPIC FINDINGS

The ducts of the periurethral glands of Skene are lined by a transitional epithelium and the glands by a columnar mucus-secreting epithelium. Periurethral cysts may be divided into four distinct types based upon their epithelial lining. Those arising from Skene's glands have a mucus-secreting columnar epithelium, which stains with mucin stain and may be associated with squamous epithelium within the cyst, thought to arise from squamous metaplasia. These cysts also have been referred to as mullerian cysts due to the similarity of the lining columnar epithelium to endocervical epithelium. These cysts are microscopically indistinguishable from mucous cysts of the vulvar vestibule.

Urothelial cysts arise from Skene's duct and are lined by transitional epithelium, although some cases near the urethral meatus may have a squamous epithelial lining. These cysts are usually encountered in infants and are rare in adults. Mesonephric cysts may occur adjacent to the urethra and are recognized by their low columnar epithelial lining, which does not stain with mucin. These cysts also have a recognizable smooth muscle layer beneath the epithelium. Keratinous (epithelial inclusion) cysts may occur adjacent to the urethra and are believed to arise from entrapped epithelium secondary to trauma or surgical procedures, although they may arise from mucous cysts or urothelial cysts as described.

DIFFERENTIAL DIAGNOSIS

The primary consideration is differentiating the Skene's duct cyst from a urethral diverticulum. Urethral diverticula are not associated with spraying of urine or diversion of the urinary stream. Patients more frequently complain of dribbling after urination and recurrent episodes of cystitis especially if the diverticular neck arises from the proximal urethra. Urethral diverticula may become infected and present as tender masses. Compressing an infected diverticulum will result in extravasation of purulent material from the distal urethra. Compression of a Skene's duct cyst results in no extravasation of fluid. The Skene's duct opens just exterior to the urethral meatus. If diagnosis is uncertain then urethroscopy may be performed; however, many diverticular cysts have such a small orifice that urethroscopy is unable to discern the opening. In such instances, double balloon pressure urethrography will be necessary to ascertain the location of the diverticular neck.

CLINICAL BEHAVIOR AND TREATMENT

The asymptomatic, small Skene's duct cyst requires no therapy other than observation. Larger cysts or expanding cysts will require excision. With a cooperative patient this may be accomplished in the office; otherwise, general or regional anesthesia will be necessary. A urethral Foley catheter may be inserted after applying 2% lidocaine gel to the urethra. This will decrease the risk of urethral injury. The area of surgery is injected with lidocaine and the epithelium overlying the cyst is then incised. The cyst wall is removed and the epithelium is reapproximated. The catheter is removed and the patient's ability to void is confirmed. Care should be exercised not to enter the urethra and create a patulous urethra or a fistula in the distal urethra, which will result in unacceptable urinary spraying. An infected Skene's duct cyst should be drained rather than excised. Excision may be performed later if the cyst is persistent. Removal of a urethral diverticulum is more appropriately performed in the operating room.

In the newborn or infant with a Skene's duct cyst large enough to be of concern (possible urinary obstruction), an effort to drain the cyst may be made by needle aspiration. If the cyst recurs, then consideration would follow for operative removal under anesthesia.

Progressive Therapeutic Options

1. Reassurance and observation, if small and asymptomatic.
2. Excision if expanding, large, or symptomatic.

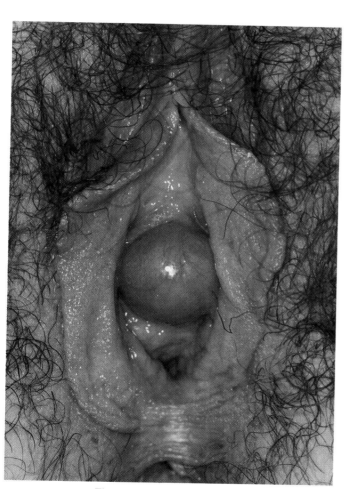

Figure 2.12. Skene's duct cyst.

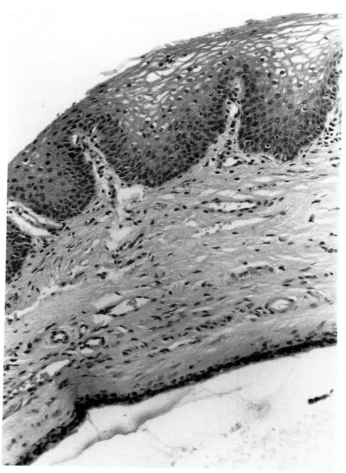

Figure 2.13. Periurethral cyst. The surface epithelium is from the distal urethra and is nonkeratinizing squamous epithelium. The periurethral cyst within the deeper tissue is lined by a flattened transitional epithelium.

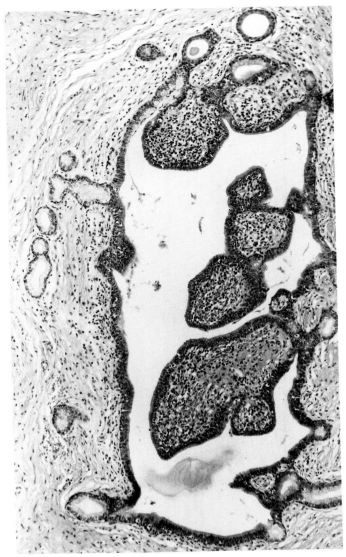

Figure 2.14. Periurethral cyst with chronic inflammation. The dilated cyst has some peripheral periurethral gland elements. A subepithelial chronic inflammatory infiltrate is present.

Vestibular Mucous Cysts

DEFINITION

Vestibular mucous cysts are simple cysts found within the vulvar vestibule that are lined by mucus-secreting columnar epithelium.

GENERAL FEATURES

Vestibular mucous cysts are cystic dilations of the minor vestibular glands located in the introitus just inferior to the hymen or hymenal remnants. These cysts are uncommon but may be seen in newborns and adults. They may be a consequence of congenital atresia of ductal openings or may result from acquired obstruction of gland openings.

CLINICAL PRESENTATION

Vestibular mucous cysts almost invariably are asymptomatic and usually are discovered upon self-examination or during routine pelvic examination. The patient who palpates the cyst is usually concerned that she has a malignancy. Although the cyst may become infected, this is exceedingly rare. A large cyst impinging upon the urethral meatus may interfere with the urinary stream and cause concern. Vestibular mucous cysts are usually discovered by the patient long before they eventuate in this difficulty.

Diagnosis of the vestibular cyst is easily accomplished by examination. The cysts are superficial and have a smooth surface. There is a translucent appearance to the superficial surface of the cyst. The cysts are mobile and nontender. Confusion with a Skene's duct cyst is possible when dealing with an anterior vestibular cyst that impinges upon the urethra.

GROSS FINDINGS

Mucous cysts are usually less than 2 cm in diameter and may be single or multiple. They typically have a blue-gray appearance, appear to be immediately beneath the epithelium, and are soft to palpation. On cut section, when formalin fixed, they contain a clear gelatinous mucoid material.

MICROSCOPIC FINDINGS

The mucous cyst has a simple mucus-secreting columnar epithelial lining that is not associated with a surrounding smooth muscle layer or inflammation. Squamous metaplastic-type epithelium may be seen adjacent to the columnar epithelium in some cysts, and complete replacement of the columnar epithelium by squamous epithelium results in the formation of a vestibular cleft. A vestibular cleft is characterized by an infolded-appearing epithelial-lined glandlike structure. The epithelium is not keratinized and is contiguous with the stratified squamous epithelium of the vestibule.

The mucus-secreting epithelium stains with mucicarmen stain, and trichrome or smooth muscle actin do not demonstrate the presence of smooth muscle about the cyst.

DIFFERENTIAL DIAGNOSIS

The clinical differentiation in this region would be between a vestibular cyst and a Skene's duct cyst. The vestibular cyst is more laterally located, although this may be difficult to discern with a large Skene's duct cyst or a large vestibular cyst. Differentiation would be moot because the therapy would be the same. A posterior vestibular cyst may be confused with a Bartholin's duct cyst, although Bartholin's duct cysts are more deeply seated. A vestibular cleft is distinguished from a keratinous cyst by its continuity with the overlying epithelium and lack of keratin or keratinous debris within the cyst.

TREATMENT

No therapy is necessary for an asymptomatic vestibular cyst. The patient may be reassured that the cyst rarely creates a problem; however, based upon the patient's wishes, the cyst may be removed easily in the clinic setting after appropriate local anesthesia. There is no need to excise a vestibular cyst noted in a newborn infant, unless there is interference with urination, in which case drainage may be accomplished by needle aspiration. Normally the cyst should be allowed to resolve spontaneously without intervention.

Progressive Therapeutic Options

1. Reassurance and observation.
2. Excision if symptomatic.

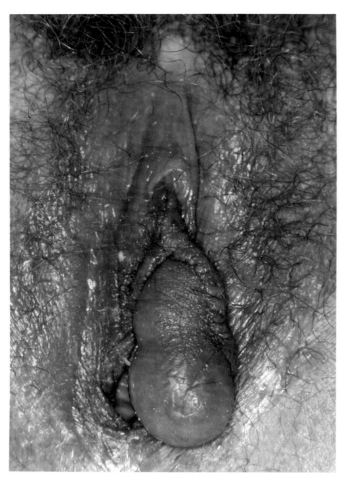

Figure 2.15. Bilobed vestibular cyst located primarily on the medial aspect of labium minus.

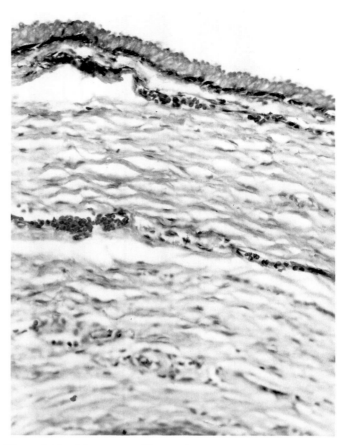

Figure 2.16. Mucous cyst. The cyst is lined by a mucus-secreting columnar epithelium. The surrounding tissue is from the vulvar vestibule and is within normal limits.

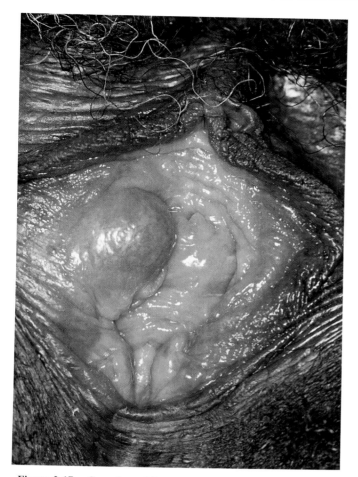

Figure 2.17. Smooth, mobile cyst present for 5 months at introitus.

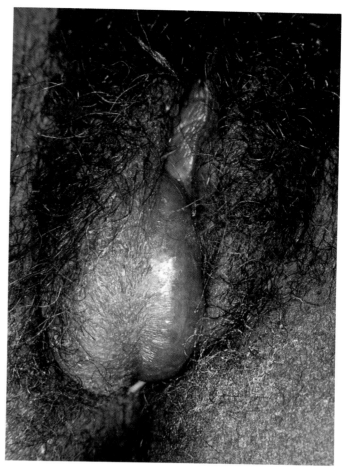

Figure 2.18. Acute-onset vulvar cyst thought to be traumatic edema and treated symptomatically without resolution. The cyst contained typical mucoid material.

3

MACULAE

MACULE ALGORITHM

MACULA (Latin maculatus: a spot): a discolored portion of skin, not elevated above surrounding tissue

Color	Presumed Diagnosis
Red	Lichen planus
	Vestibulitis
Dark	Lentigo simplex
	Melanosis vulvae
Hypopigmented	Lichen sclerosus
	Vitiligo

Figure 3.1. Macule algorithm.

Lichen Planus

DEFINITION

Lichen planus is an inflammatory disease of unknown etiology that may involve skin and mucosal surfaces.

GENERAL FEATURES

It is uncommon to see a patient with lichen planus in a gynecologic practice. More frequently these patients will present to dermatologists for evaluation of their papular skin lesions or to oral surgeons and dentists for evaluation of their desquamative and ulcerative buccal lesions.

CLINICAL PRESENTATION

With involvement of the vagina the patient may complain of uncomfortable intercourse and a sen-

sation that vaginal depth is diminishing. There may be a vaginal discharge, which may be tinged with blood. Questioning the patient who presents with these symptoms about skin or oral lesions is usually informative. Physical examination may reveal the presence of oral lesions, which may be present without symptoms. Patients also may complain of hair loss. There may also be a history of papular lesions on skin surfaces (ankles, dorsal surfaces of the hands, and flexor surfaces of the wrists and forearms). These may be pruritic.

Although lichen planus is an uncommon disease, it should be considered in the differential diagnosis of desquamative vaginitis. It typically involves the vestibule and vagina. The vestibule may demonstrate a reticular pattern, known as Wickham's striae. The vagina may be markedly erythematous and a serosanguinous discharge may be present. With progressive disease, the walls of the vagina may adhere to one another and the vaginal vault may be lost. As with lichen sclerosus, vulvar architecture may be obscured with fusion of the labia minora and labia majora, resulting in obliteration of the clitoris. It is feasible to misdiagnose lichen planus as lichen sclerosus. Lichen sclerosus patients do not have reticular patterns in the vestibule and typically do not have a desquamative vaginitis. To evaluate the patient completely one must perform a careful general dermatologic review, including examination of the scalp and the oral mucous membranes. The occurrence of the typical papular lesions on the skin and the reticular pattern in the mouth would further support a diagnosis of lichen planus. Ultimately biopsy will be the most definitive method of arriving at the appropriate diagnosis. Biopsies are most productive when taken from intact skin or mucous membranes. Ulcerative lesions are difficult to assess histologically and will demonstrate inflammation. A biopsy from a reticulate lesion at the vestibule will be most helpful and is readily obtained.

MICROSCOPIC FINDINGS

Lichen planus (LP) may have a variety of histopathologic features within the vulva, depending upon whether or not the LP involves hair-bearing keratinized skin, or non-hair-bearing, nonkeratinized vulvar vestibule.

Within hair-bearing and keratinized epithelium, LP is characterized by a lichenoid interface chronic inflammatory cell infiltrate, which consists predominantly of lymphocytes without plasma cells. The inflammation is lichenoid in that it involves the superficial dermis, immediately beneath the epithelium, and extends into the basalar and parabasalar epithelium. The basal epithelial cells have liquification necrosis; colloid bodies are present secondary to degeneration of keratinocytes. The inflammatory infiltrate obscures the interface at the epidermal-dermal junction. The epithelium may have prominent acanthosis with a prominent granular layer and hyperkeratosis. In older lesions, acanthosis may be absent and the epithelium thinned with loss of the rete ridges. Ulceration and bullae may occur in severe lesions.

When LP involves the nonkeratinized epithelium of the vestibule, the interface inflammatory infiltrate is present; however, the inflammatory cell population may contain plasma cells within the predominantly lymphocytic infiltrate. Thinning of the epithelium, with inflammatory cell exocytosis, is common. Hyperkeratosis and a prominent granular layer usually are not present. Colloid bodies with keratinocyte liquification necrosis, bullae, and ulceration are evident in severe cases. Silver and periodic acid-Schiff stains for bacteria, fungi, and spirochetes are negative.

ADJUNCTIVE STUDIES

Indirect and direct immunohistology may be necessary for confirmation of diagnosis if the possibility of pemphigus or pemphigoid exists. Pemphigus and pemphigoid (most commonly cicatricial pemphigoid) may result in desquamative changes in the vagina and should be included in the differential diagnosis of desquamative vaginitis. Interestingly, lichen planus and bullous pemphigoid may occur in the same patient.

CLINICAL BEHAVIOR AND TREATMENT

The management of patients with vulvovaginal lichen planus is difficult. The mainstay of therapy consists of topical application of low- to moderate-strength steroid preparations. These preparations are applied readily to the vulvar and vestibular regions but intravaginal insertion poses a problem. Rectal suppositories such as Cort-Dome with 25 mg of hydrocortisone may be inserted into the vagina once or twice daily for control of vaginal symptoms. However, most patients do not experience significant long-term response to intravaginal steroids. The vaginal vault will continue to scar. To keep the vault open and prevent adhesions it will be necessary, in selected cases, to use vaginal dilators. Vaginal maintenance may be accomplished with daily use of Lucite dilators and the therapeutic response may be augmented by sitting on an Ingram's bicycle seat daily with the Lucite dilator in the vagina. The dilator may be lubricated with a hydrocortisone cream. Most patients will be unable to maintain this rigorous regimen. Anecdotal reports concerning the successful use of oral griseofulvin, 250 mg twice a day, should warrant a trial of this rather innocuous medication. Etretinate (Tegison) has been used to ameliorate oral lichen planus; however, discontinuation of the medication results in recurrence of the oral lesions. Long-term use of retinoids may result in liver dysfunction and there is no documented successful use of retinoids for vulvovaginal lichen planus. Immunosuppressant therapy with cyclosporine has been used to manage oral lichen planus, either as a mouthwash or administered systemically. Although success has been noted with immunosuppressant therapy, recurrence of the disease has been reported after discontinuation of immunosuppression. Dapsone, a pharmacologic agent used to treat leprosy, has on occasion demonstrated ameliorative effect and may be considered, but only after performing a screen for glucose-6-phosphate dehydrogenase (G6PD) deficiency. Patients with G6PD deficiency may develop a profound anemia when exposed to Dapsone. Patients treated with Dapsone should be observed closely for evidence of anemia (weekly complete blood cell counts). Dosage is 50–100 mg daily.

Progressive Therapeutic Options

1. Topical steroids
   (a) Betamethasone valerate 0.1% (Valisone) ointment to vulva.
   (b) Hydrocortisone 25 mg (Cort-Dome) suppository every day in vagina; augment with vaginal dilators to maintain vault patency. If low-potency suppositories are ineffective, try a short course of vaginal 0.1% betamethasone cream daily (2 weeks).
2. Consider trial of Griseofulvin 250 mg orally twice a day.
3. Consider trial of Dapsone 50–100 mg orally every day after negative G6PD screen. (follow complete blood cell counts closely).
4. Consider isotretinoin (Accutane) 0.5–1 mg/kg/day in two divided doses
   or
   etretinate (Tegison) 0.75–1 mg/kg/day in two divided doses
   (a) Monitor liver function tests, cholesterol, triglycerides, and complete blood cell counts.
   (b) Counsel concerning teratogenicity and need for optimum contraception.
5. Consider cyclosporine 1 mg/kg/day (may increase by increments of 0.5 mg/kg/day every 2–4 weeks to maximum of 3–5 mg/kg/day)
   (a) Monitor complete blood cell counts, liver function tests, cholesterol, triglyceride, electrolytes, urea nitrogen, creatinine, creatinine clearance.
   (b) Counsel concerning risks of renal compromise and possibility of future development of neoplasia.
   (c) **USE REQUIRES DISEASE SEVERITY SUFFICIENT TO WARRANT RISKS.**

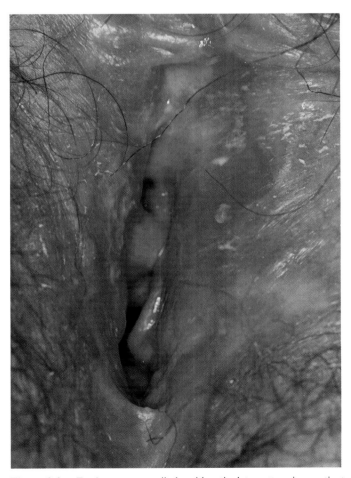

Figure 3.2. Erythematous vestibule with reticulate pattern in a patient complaining of burning and occasional bleeding. Biopsy was consistent with lichen planus and patient was managed with Valisone 0.1% ointment.

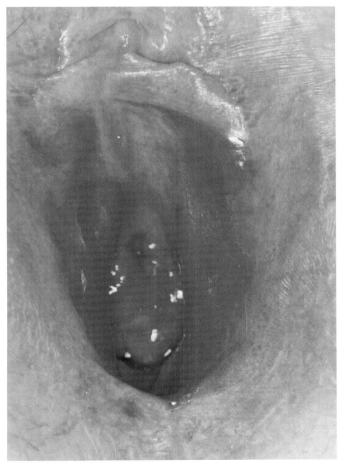

Figure 3.3. Lichen planus in a patient with dyspareunia for 8 months. Condition involved vagina and vestibule. Acute vaginal occlusion necessitated vaginal dilators (candlesticks) and topical steroids (Cort-Dome suppositories).

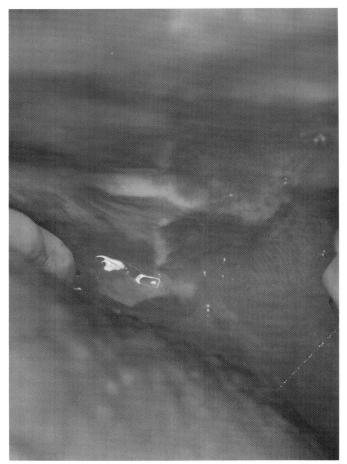

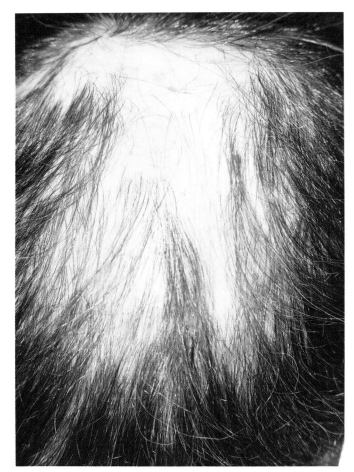

Figure 3.4. Reticular buccal mucosa lesion in a patient with vulvovaginal lichen planus.

Figure 3.5. Alopecia in patient with oral and vulvovaginal lichen planus.

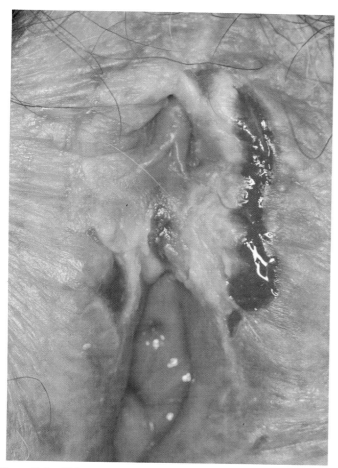

Figure 3.6. Velvety plaque-like lesions suggestive of plasma cell vulvitis in a patient with lichen planus. After 3 months of Temovate ointment, lesions resolved.

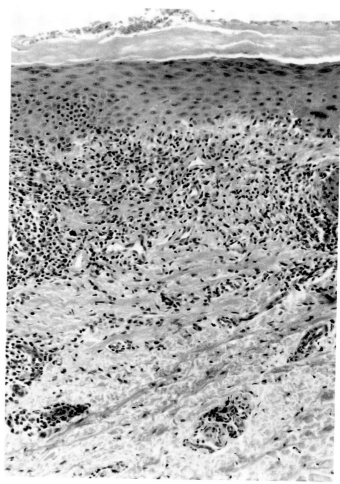

Figure 3.7. Lichen planus. The epithelium is keratinized and has a spongiotic basal layer. There is a marked interface inflammatory infiltrate consisting primarily of lymphocytes without plasma cells.

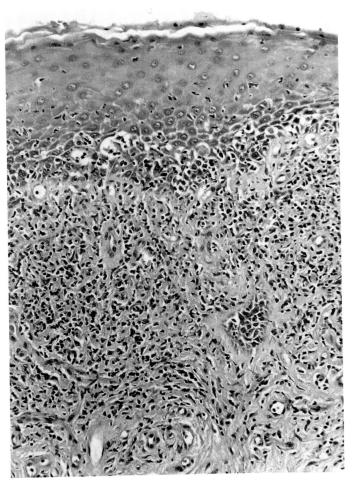

Figure 3.8. Lichen planus. The interface inflammation obscures the epithelial stromal junction.

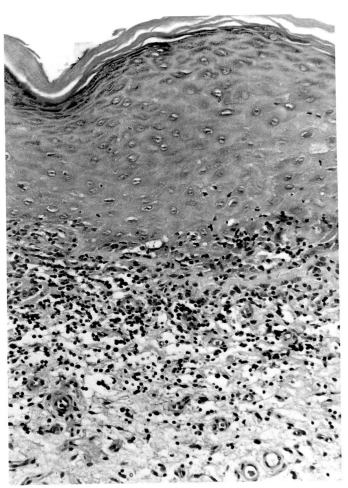

Figure 3.9. Lichen planus. The epithelium is slightly hyperkeratotic. A prominent interface inflammatory cell infiltrate is present, which consists predominately of lymphocytes without plasma cells and obscures the basal layer and its junction with the underlying dermis.

Lichen Sclerosus

DEFINITION

Lichen sclerosus is a chronic dermatologic condition associated with epithelial thinning, distinctive dermal changes, and inflammation (Table 3.1).

GENERAL FEATURES

The prevalence of lichen sclerosus is unknown; however, it is one of the most common conditions treated in vulvar clinics. Likewise the etiology is unknown, although various mechanisms have been proposed, including immunologic, genetic, androgen receptor inactivity or deficiency, and epidermal growth factor deficiency.

CLINICAL PRESENTATION

Most commonly, patients present in the peri-menopausal and postmenopausal years complaining of vulvar pruritus. Occasionally patients may complain of burning and painful intercourse. Lichen sclerosus may present throughout the reproductive spectrum and symptoms may be observed as early as 6 months of age. Although the disease may be noted in other regions of the body, the vulva is the most common site in women. On examination, the typical patient with lichen sclerosus will demonstrate thin, white skin, localized to the labia minora and/or labia majora. The condition may extend to the perineal body and between the gluteal folds and have a symmetrical distribution. If the patient is seen early in the course of her disease, biopsy may demonstrate minimal epitheleal change or inflammation. As the disease progresses there will be loss of the normal vulvar architecture, with loss of the distinction between the labia majora and minora and loss of the clitoral hood. Eventually the clitoris will be covered by the fusing labia. Shrinkage of the introitus and perineal area may result in painful intercourse and may preclude intercourse. Unlike lichen planus, the vagina is not involved. Painful defecation and bleeding with defecation due to splitting of the involved skin may occur. Intense pruritis causes scratching with resultant excoriation of skin. Perhaps as a consequence of this trauma, areas of lichen sclerosus may become hyperplastic. These areas of hyperplastic epithelium within fields of lichen sclerosus are believed to be at risk for the development of squamous cell carcinoma. Although lichen sclerosus is not considered to be a premalignant condition, areas of hyperplastic epithelium occurring within fields of lichen sclerosus may be sites of premalignant or malignant change.

MICROSCOPIC FINDINGS

The microscopic features of lichen sclerosus are variable and are related primarily to the age of the process and the degree of secondary changes related to rubbing or scratching. The characteristic features include loss of rete ridges; a homogenous appearance to the superficial dermis with associated edema, fibrin, and apparent decrease in collagen and vascularity. A chronic inflammatory infiltrate is present immediately beneath the edematous overlying dermis. The epithelium may be markedly thinned, eroded, or ulcerated; however, the epithelium can be markedly thickened with a thickly keratinized surface. Some spongiosis is commonly seen, especially involving the basalar epithelial cells, where vacuolar degeneration may be seen. These basalar changes may be associated with separation of the overlying epithelium from the underlying dermis with focal bullous changes. These changes may be so severe as to resemble a bullous disease. Blood may be present within the superficial dermis and immediately beneath the epithelium, forming small hematomas. Ulceration and bleeding are usually secondary to rubbing. The degree of superficial dermal edema can be highly variable, with little edema present in early changes and marked edema in the fully evolved case. Old lesions may have minimal edematous features and appear sclerotic. With advanced lesions, associated with shrinkage and fibrosis of the vulva, it may be very difficult or impossible to separate these findings from advanced lichen planus or scleroderma (morphea). The chronic inflammatory infiltrate may be minimal in early lesions and severe in a fully involved lesion. The inflammatory infiltrate consists predominately of lymphocytes; however, secondary infection from prior recent biopsies or localized trauma can result in an acute inflammatory infiltrate or other associated changes.

Table 3.1
Classification of Vulvar Nonneoplastic Epithelial Disorders: International Society for the Study of Vulvar Disease

1972–1986	1987
Lichen sclerosus	Lichen sclerosus
Hyperplastic dystrophy	Squamous cell hyperplasia
Mixed dystrophy	Other dermatoses

From Ridley CM, Frankman D, Jones IS, et al. Hum Pathol 1989; 20:495–496.

DIFFERENTIAL DIAGNOSIS

Diagnosis is suspected upon noting the symmetric parchmentlike white epithelium of lichen sclerosus. Vitiligo may be confused with this condition, but the skin in patients with vitiligo does not appear to be atrophic. Another condition that may mimic lichen sclerosus is lichen planus. Lichen planus may eventuate in loss of vulvar architecture, as does lichen sclerosus. However, lichen planus typically has an erosive vaginal component and a reticulate pattern at the introitus.

When lichen sclerosus results in self-induced trauma from scratching, the ability to diagnose the condition clinically becomes markedly diminished. Palpation must be combined with visualization in assessing these patients. Any area of hyperplastic epithelium or erosive disease should be biopsied to evalute for evidence of squamous cell carcinoma. Hyperplastic erosive vulvitis associated with lichen sclerosus may resemble vulvar Paget's disease. When dealing with patients with lichen sclerosus, close follow-up will be necessary over the course of years to assess for these changes and any suspicion for malignancy. There is a recognized lifetime risk of vulvar carcinoma in these women which may be 3–5% or higher.

ADJUNCTIVE STUDIES

Consider thyroid function studies because perhaps one-third of patients with lichen sclerosus also have hypothyroidism. (This is not a causal relationship.)

CLINICAL BEHAVIOR AND TREATMENT

The therapy for lichen sclerosus, properly evaluated, without evidence of neoplasm, consists of an initial effort to control pruritus. This will usually necessitate the use of medium potency steroid ointment such as betamethasone valerate 0.1% (Valisone). Steroidal creams do not appear to be as efficacious as ointments in the management of vulvar pruritus. It will usually be necessary to apply the steroidal ointment 2–3 times daily for 2 weeks to control pruritus. At this point patients may often terminate steroidal ointments and use them only episodically with the onset of pruritus. The continued prolonged use of medium- or high-potency steroid ointment may result in thinning of vulvar skin outside of the field of lichen sclerosus and the potential for subsequent steroid-induced atrophy and fragile vulvar skin. If possible, low-potency steroids such as hydrocortisone may be used after initial clinical success with medium- to high-potency steroids.

For patients with hyperplastic lesions of the vulva in whom biopsies have excluded neoplastic changes and in whom medium-strength steroids have failed to alleviate pruritus, superpotent steroids may be used for short intervals. Halobetasol (Ultravate) and clobetasol (Temovate) ointment may provide remarkable resolution of hyperplastic epithelium when used in this manner. Usually, lower potency steroid ointments are used as maintenance therapy; however, the long-term use of topical high-potency corticosteroids applied 1–3 times per week at night has proved effective in persistent cases. Occasionally it will be necessary to inject regions of lichen sclerosus that are unresponsive to topical applications with intralesional steroids such as Kenalog-10. This can be accomplished in the clinic setting.

Perhaps the most commonly used topical preparation in the United States for lichen sclerosus is 2% testosterone proprionate in petrolatum. This topical preparation is applied 2–3 times per day for up to 6 months. After completion of the initial phase of therapy, frequency of application may be reduced based upon response and side effects. Side effects may be fairly significant in some patients. There may be complaints of clitoromegaly, resulting in clitorial discomfort. Occasionally patients will complain of burning, and erythema will be noted in the vulvar skin. Rarely hirsutism may be observed. These untoward side effects may result in discontinuation of the topical application of testosterone. It is preferable, when using testosterone in patients with pruritus, to alleviate the pruritus with topical steroids before initiating testosterone therapy. Patients should be informed that testosterone therapy will be lifelong. In the authors' practice, testosterone preparations are no longer used. Steroid preparations applied topically are the preferred approach.

For children with lichen sclerosus, testosterone has the potential for masculinizing the external genitalia and a more appropriate therapeutic agent is topical progesterone. Topical progesterone may be prepared by mixing 400 mg of progesterone in oil with 4 oz of aquaphor and applying this twice daily. Once again, it may be necessary to use topical steroids to control pruritus before beginning the topical progesterone applications in young children. Topical corticosteroids alone may be sufficient therapy. Topical progesterone may also be used in adults who do not respond to steroids or testosterone.

It may be occasionally necessary to excise hyperplastic or fissured areas of lichen sclerosus that are unresponsive to the previously mentioned regimens. Patients must be forewarned that there is a high recurrence rate of lichen sclerosus after excision. Skin grafting has been attempted to manage patients with lichen sclerosus; however, lichen sclerosus may recur in the grafted skin.

It should be reemphasized that although managing patients with lichen sclerosus is often gratifying, these patients need careful follow-up. Regular visits should be scheduled at approximately 3–6-month intervals for patients without evidence of hyperplasia to rule out the development of hyperplastic lesions. Patients with hyperplastic lesions should be seen more frequently, perhaps at 3-month intervals, and failure of lesions to regress with high-potency steroid therapy should prompt biopsy to rule out the development of neoplasia. In many instances these biopsies can be excisional biopsies, with complete removal of the hyperplastic lesion.

A final note should be made concerning the use of emollients. Lichen sclerosus is a condition that typically presents as thin, parchmentlike skin, a poor barrier to the loss of moisture. Although steroid preparations may diminish the inflammatory response within the skin, they will not correct the underlying condition. An effort should be made by the patient to avoid excessive drying of this skin after showering or bathing. Moisturizing compounds may be applied, but often the simple application of a thin layer of Vaseline may improve moisture retention and diminish the necessity to resort frequently to the use of steroid-containing ointments.

Progressive Therapeutic Options

1. To control pruritis in nonhyperplastic skin, apply betamethasone valerate 0.1% ointment twice daily for 2–3 weeks and then taper use or use a less potent steroidal ointment. Maintain moisture content of skin with a thin layer of moisturizing lotions, creams, or ointments.
2. To control pruritis in hyperplastic skin, after biopsy excludes malignancy, consider short-term application of highly potent steroids, halobetasol (Ultravate) 0.05% (or) clobetasol (Temovate) 0.05% ointment twice a day. Taper use after 2–3 weeks and consider medium- or low-potency steroid ointments for long-term use.
3. For pruritis unresponsive to topical steroids, inject triamcinolone (Kenalog-10) at 1-cm grids.

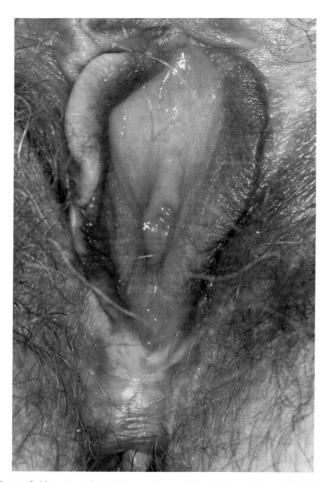

Figure 3.10. A patient with pruritus and classic hypopigmented lichen sclerosus.

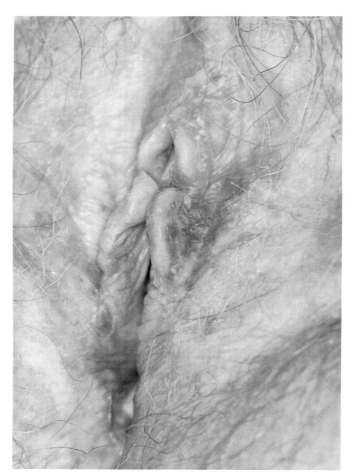

Figure 3.11. Excoriation due to scratching. Biopsy confirmed lichen sclerosus. Testosterone had been of no benefit; however, topical Valisone 0.1% ointment resolved pruritus.

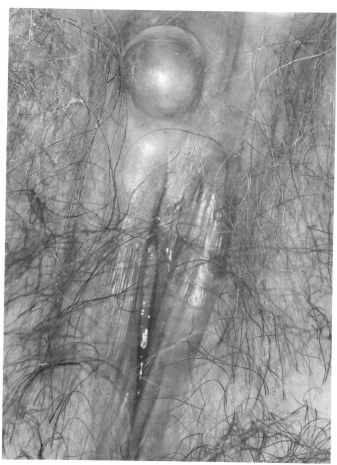

Figure 3.12. Clitoromegaly developing in a patient with lichen sclerosus after 18 months of topical testosterone.

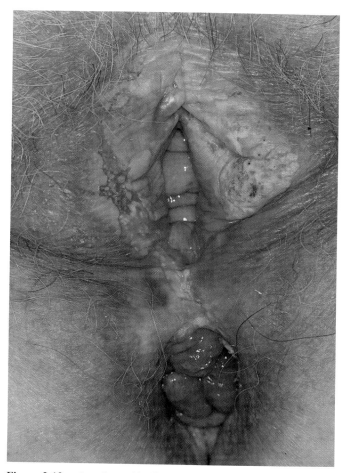

Figure 3.13. A patient with 12-year history of lichen sclerosus treated with testosterone and Valisone. Biopsies of right and left labia demonstrated lichen sclerosus with marked hyperkeratosis and hyperparakeratosis. Within 12 months patient will develop superficially invasive carcinoma of left labium managed by wide local excision.

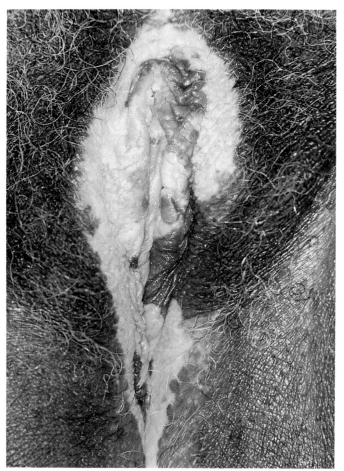

Figure 3.14. An asymptomatic woman with hypertrophic lichen sclerosus on biopsies of right periclitoral and right labial skin. Patient was managed with Valisone 0.1% ointment. Note diffuse changes consistent with vitiligo.

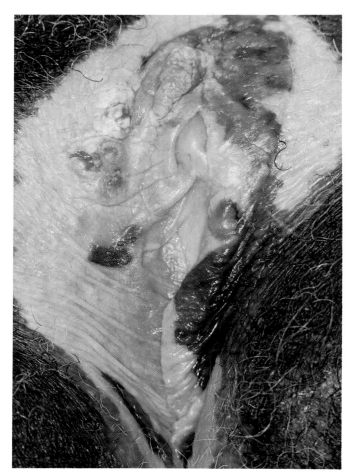

Figure 3.15. Five months later, the patient in Figure 3.14 returned with complaint of pruritus. Biopsy of right periclitoral area demonstrated invasive squamous cell carcinoma. Wide local excision demonstrated 3.2-mm invasion, and groin node dissection was negative.

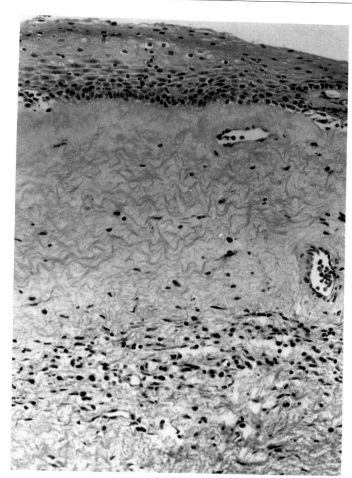 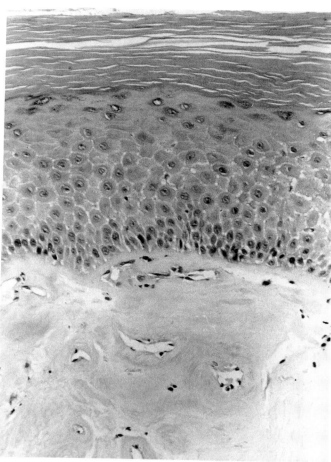

Figure 3.16. Lichen sclerosus. The epithelium is thinly keratinized and markedly thinned in this advanced case. Prominent superficial dermal homogenization is present. A bandlike, predominately lymphocytic, inflammatory infiltrate is seen below the involved edematous dermis.

Figure 3.17. Lichen sclerosis. High magnification demonstrates marked hyperkeratosis in this case. The epithelium is thinned and spongiotic. Thin-walled sclerotic vessels are present within the edematous dermis.

Lentigo Simplex and Melanosis Vulvae

DEFINITION

Lentigo simplex is a hyperpigmented macular lesion resulting from a localized excess production of melanin by melanocytes. Melanocytes may be increased in number within the basal layer of the epithelium.

GENERAL FEATURES

Most commonly seen in older women, lentigo will be a frequent finding in vulvar clinics.

CLINICAL PRESENTATION

Rarely, patients will present after self-examination, complaining of hyperpigmented lesions in vulvar or vestibular epithelium. More commonly the lesions will be discovered by the examining physician during routine gynecologic examination. Lesions are frequently multiple, have somewhat irregular borders, and are flat. Size may vary from 1 to 4 mm. The color is usually a shade of brown. Lesions may be present on the labia majora, labia minora, and in the vestibule. Similar lesions may be present in extra-genital skin. Lentigo is differentiated from freckles by a lack of response (hyperpigmentation) to sunlight exposure. Pigmented areas larger than 4 mm with the histologic findings of lentigo simplex are referred to as vulvar melanosis. Areas of vulvar melanosis may be large, exceeding 10 cm in diameter.

The diagnosis of lentigo simplex is easily suspected after visual inspection. Given the inability to confirm this diagnosis absolutely without histologic assay, it is preferred to perform an excisional biopsy and obtain histologic confirmation of the diagnosis. Histologic examination will exclude atypical nevi and melanoma. The patient's anxiety will be allayed and the physician will be more comfortable with the clinical assessment.

MICROSCOPIC FINDINGS

The epithelium of lentigo simplex is typically slightly hyperplastic with acanthosis and slight clubbing of the rete ridges. Hyperpigmentation is evident, predominantly in the basal and parabasal areas, although pigmentation may be extensive. The melanin pigment is evident as granules within the keratinocytes. Functioning melanocytes are present within the epithelium near the basement membrane; however, nevomelanocytic nests and Pagetoid growth are not present. Within the superficial dermis, a mild inflammatory cell infiltrate may be present. The microscopic findings of vulvar lentigo simplex and vulvar melanosis essentially lack distinguishing features other than for size.

CLINICAL BEHAVIOR AND TREATMENT

Excisional biopsy is both the diagnostic and therapeutic approach to lentigo simplex on the vulva and vestibule. For patients with multiple lentigines, excisional biopsies should be prioritized to those areas with markedly irregular borders and marked hyperpigmentation.

Progressive Therapeutic Option

1. Excisional biopsy for confirmation of diagnosis.

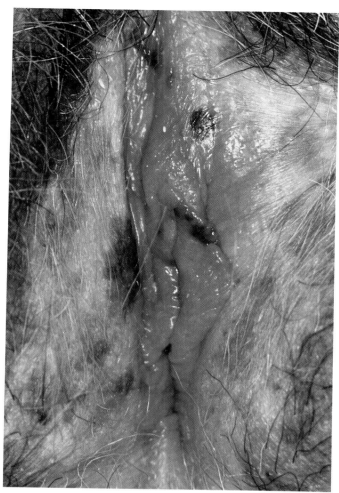

Figure 3.18. Multiple hyperpigmented lesions of typical lentigo simplex and melanosis.

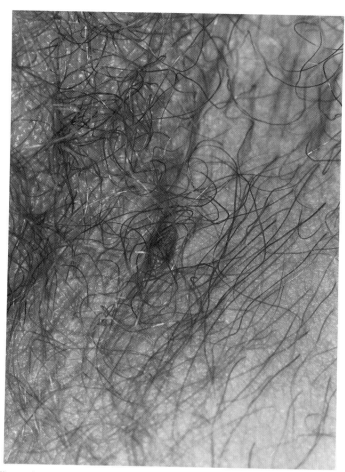

Figure 3.19. Evaluated lesion believed to be compound nevus. Biopsy demonstrated lentigo simplex.

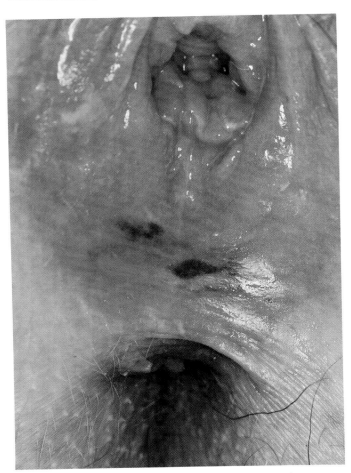

Figure 3.20. Diffuse changes of melanosis at introitus.

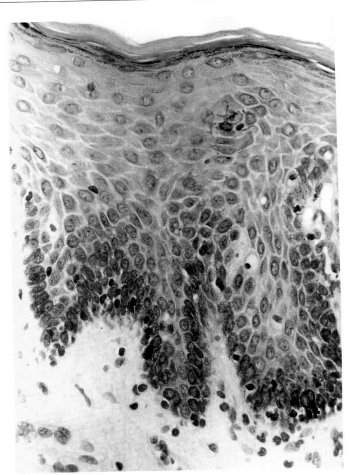

Figure 3.21. Lentigo simplex. Pigmented keratinocytes and melanocytes are evident within the basal layer. The epithelium is neither thickened nor hyperkeratotic in this case. A few lymphocytes are present in the superficial dermis.

Vestibulitis

DEFINITION

Vulvar vestibulitis is a chronic, painful, inflammatory process of the vulvar vestibule characterized by pain within the vestibule, entry dyspareunia, and erythema within the vestibule. The erythema is most prominently noted about the minor vestibular gland openings.

GENERAL FEATURES

The etiology of vulvar vestibulitis is unknown. Although the frequency is considered to be low, increasing numbers of patients appear to be afflicted with this disabling condition.

CLINICAL PRESENTATION

Patients will present with complaints of dyspareunia. Age at presentation may range from 19 to 81 years of age, with a median of 36 years. Most patients will have been sexually active for 12–14 years before the onset of their dyspareunia. Most patients will have used tampons and will have used them for 10–12 years before onset of symptoms. The most common symptom is painful intercourse. The pain is usually described as a burning pain. Approximately 33% of patients will also complain of the inability to insert tampons. Intercourse will frequently be so painful as to preclude intromission. Symptoms may be present for 1–55 years. The usual duration of symptoms will be 2–5 years. The pain that is noted with intercourse is present at the introitus. It is not a deep dyspareunia. It usually begins with foreplay or intromission and persists for hours to days after intercourse.

Diagnosis is almost invariably suspected after obtaining the distraught patient's history. The patient should be involved in the examination process and this is easily accomplished by providing her with a mirror so that she might visualize the vestibule as it is examined. The vestibule should be examined before insertion of a vaginal speculum. Most commonly, erythema will be noted in a horseshoe-shaped distribution extending from the midvestibule posteriorly to the contralateral side of the vestibule. Often the Bartholin's gland ducts will appear as inflamed, prominent openings. Occasionally the inflammation will extend about the posterior-lateral periclitoral region. A cotton swab applied gently to the vestibule will elicit intense discomfort. The level of discomfort will often appear to be out of proportion to the clinical findings. The region of tenderness should be mapped carefully. Colposcopic examination of the vestibule should then be accomplished after application of 3% acetic acid. The patient should be forewarned that this will cause burning. Vestibular epithelium may be diffusely slightly aceto-white; however, aceto-white epithelium alone or in association with squamous papillomatosis should warrant consideration for biopsy. Notation of changes in the histologic specimen consistent with human papillomavirus may have potentially significant implications for therapeutic approaches. It is uncommon to find these human papillomavirus changes in the vestibule in patients with vestibulitis. Molecular biologic techniques for detection of papillomavirus may be of value in controversial cases. At the completion of the colposcopic examination, the acetic acid should be lavaged with normal saline. It is often appropriate at this point to apply lidocaine gel or ointment to the vestibule to accomplish the vaginal examination and to determine whether or not the patient may have a therapeutic response to the application of such a preparation. The vagina should then be examined for evidence of vaginitis. Frequently patients will give a history of chronic and recurrent yeast infections, although it is uncommon in the vestibulitis patient to find evidence of such an infection. A wet preparation of vaginal secretions should be obtained. Evidence of yeast infection or bacterial vaginosis should be documented.

MICROSCOPIC FINDINGS

The pathologic findings of vulvar vestibulitis include submucosal superficial chronic inflammation which consists predominately of lymphocytes, and approximately three-quarters of the cases will also have plasma cells present. Minor vestibular glands are seen in about one-third of the specimens and, when present, the inflammation is typically within the submucosa surrounding the gland and usually does not involve the glandular epithelium. The overlying epithelium of the vestibule may appear thinned, and some inflammatory cells may be seen within the epithelium, essentially identical to that of the vagina or ectocervix. This glycogen-rich epithelium or spongiosis should not be confused with koilocytosis associated with human papillomavirus (HPV) effect. HPV infection, related to HPV types 6,11,16, or 18, is uncommon in vestibulitis and is identified in approximately 10% of cases. If HPV infection is present, there is usually typical koilocystosis, with enlarged nuclei, which are larger than the underlying basal cell nuclei. In addition, there is usually parabasalar hyperplasia, dyskeratosis, parakeratosis and multinucleation of the keratinocytes. Studies searching for HPV in the specimen, using in situ hybridization or polymerase-chain reaction, are of value in resolving equivocal cases.

CLINICAL BEHAVIOR AND TREATMENT

No therapy has been uniformly successful in managing vestibulitis. Although human papillomavirus has been associated with vestibulitis symptoms, it is not known to be a cause of vestibulitis. Human papillomavirus may have such a high background prevalence in the population in general that its observance in the lower reproductive tract in a patient with vestibulitis may not reflect a causal relationship. However, patients with evidence of human papillomavirus may be treated successfully with interferon injections. Success rates with these injections have varied but are probably in the range of 50–60%. Additional injections may be necessary for recurrence of the patient's symptoms. These injections are given on Mondays, Wednesdays, and Fridays for 4 successive weeks. The vestibule is treated as a clock face and each hour designation will receive 1 million units of injected interferon. One million units of interferon will be injected on each of the 12 injection days and at the completion of 4 weeks of therapy each hour designation will have received one injection. Patients are forewarned that flu-like symptoms may be noted during the course of therapy. A therapeutic response may not occur for 1–3 months after completion of the injections. These injections should not be given to pregnant women and patients are advised to refrain from intercourse during the period of injections.

For most vestibulitis patients, no evidence of human papillomavirus will be noted. The management of these patients is an enigma. Many regimens have been attempted. Topical steroid creams invariably have failed to alleviate discomfort. Likewise topical anesthetics used alone almost invariably have failed to alleviate discomfort. Other modalities that have been attempted without significant therapeutic response include alcohol injections, Dapsone, nonsteroidal antiinflammatory drugs, Zovirax, steroid injections, and trichloroacetic acid. A rare patient has responded to Zostrix applications. Zostrix is a chili-pepper derivative used to treat patients with herpes zoster neuralgia. It is most uncomfortable when applied to the vestibule and will usually require narcotic analgesia to accomplish application.

The cream should be applied 4–5 times daily for 1 week and then tapered over successive weeks. Patients should be forewarned that the discomfort may be intense and that the success rate for therapy is low. Alcohol injections are not of value and should be avoided. They may exacerbate the condition and result in ulceration of the vestibule.

Given the lack of understanding concerning the etiology of vestibulitis, it should perhaps be treated as a chronic pain state. Often noted is the extreme degree of anxiety and high stress level in patients with vestibulitis. For chronic pain conditions, the use of tricyclic antidepressants such as amitriptyline has demonstrated significant amelioration of pain perception. Dosaging of amitriptyline (Elavil) is usually started at a low level, 10 mg three times a day because patients will often note drowsiness at work on the higher dosages. It may be necessary to increase the dose to higher levels such as 25 mg three times a day but this should be accomplished gradually. In addition to the tricyclic antidepressant therapy, topical applications of lidocaine (5% Xylocaine ointment or 2% lidocaine gel) may be used to augment the benefit. Occasionally patients will notice burning associated with topical use of lidocaine preparations and they must be discontinued. Patients should also be warned that the sexual partner may experience localized anesthesia secondary to contact with these preparations. Topical anesthetics will not cure the problem but on occasion may allow intromission to be accomplished.

Mechanical efforts to alleviate the discomfort should begin with questioning concerning penile size and a comparison to the patient's introital diameter. Often couples will note a significant disparity between the size of the erect penis and the introitus. Introital dilatation may be necessary since many patients are nulliparous. Introital dilatation may be accomplished with dilators, which may range from inexpensive candlesticks to more expensive Lucite dilators.

Interventional therapy consists of laser surgery and surgical excision. Pulse dye laser surgery may be successful, although surgical excision of the vestibule (vestibulectomy) has been more widely utilized. This operation should be reserved for those patients who have failed to respond to previous attempts to control their discomfort. Careful counseling should be accomplished before performing the vestibulectomy. This operation will be temporarily disabling and will be expensive. The success rate for the operation is approximately 50–60%. Before the vestibulectomy the area of tenderness should be outlined carefully and adequate margins should be obtained to ensure excision of the area of inflammation. The perineal skin and the vaginal epithelium should be undermined to obtain mobilization after removal of the vestibule. If this is not accomplished, breakdown of the excision site is likely. Hemostasis should be meticulous. In the patient with a size-discrepant introitus it may be necessary to accomplish introital widening during the surgery. In accomplishing this, care should be taken not to disrupt the levator ani function.

Regardless of the mode used to treat vulvar vestibulitis patients, careful and thorough counseling should be accomplished. These patients will require a great deal of time and their management will often be frustrating to both the patient and physician. Local support groups for vestibulitis patients may augment the management.

Progressive Therapeutic Options

1. Interferon injections for HPV-associated vestibulitis. One million units per injection site (total of 12 injection sites), given over the course of 4 weeks. Interferon concentration recommended is 3 million units/mL. Inject on Mondays, Wednesdays, and Fridays. Total injected is 12 million units to entire introitus. Injection sites are within the vestibule (superimposed clock face).
2. Vaginal dilators for size discrepant introitus. Use of introital lubricant during intercourse.
3. Topical lidocaine (5% Xylocaine ointment or 2% lidocaine gel).
4. Amitriptyline (Elavil) 10–25 mg orally three times a day (start with a low dose).
5. Vestibulectomy after appropriate counseling (50–60% success rate).

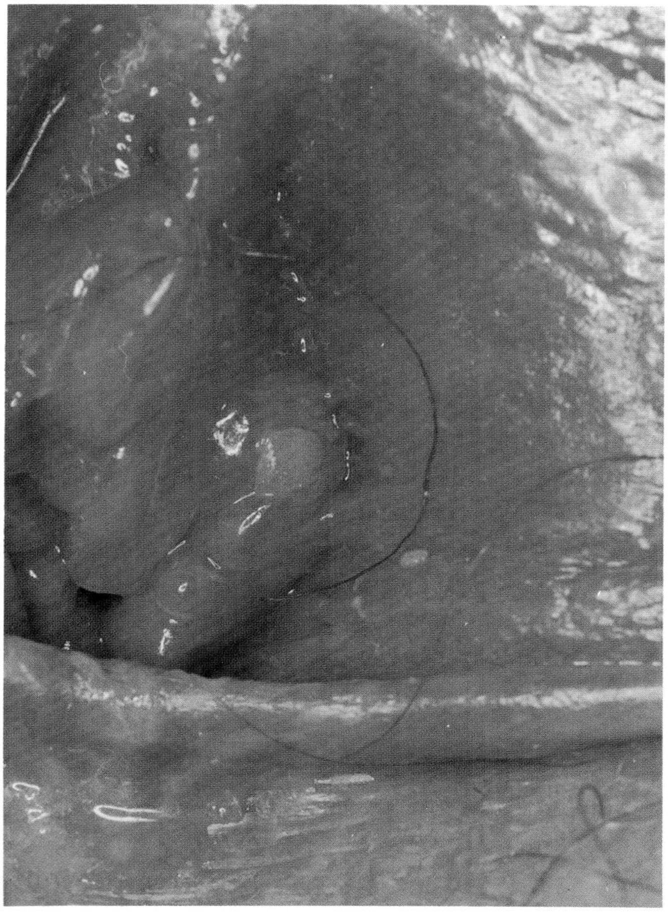

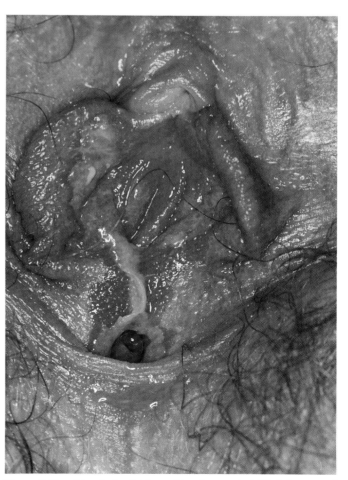

Figure 3.22. Aceto-white epithelium in a patient with severe dyspareunia. Management with interferon injections for 4 weeks resulted in resolution of symptoms.

Figure 3.23. Chemical vulvitis resulting from topical 5% 5-fluorouracil vestibulitis. Vestibulitis symptoms persisted after resolution of chemical reaction.

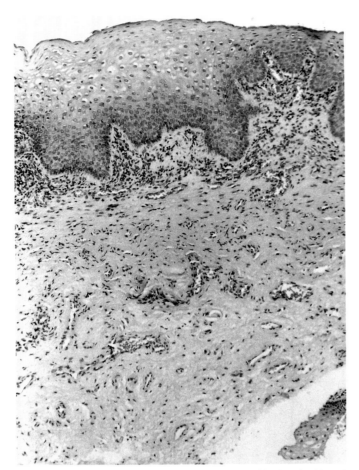

Figure 3.24. Vulvar vestibulitis. The vestibular epithelium is thinned in one area, with prominent vessels within the mucosal papillae and underlying the epithelium. The inflammatory infiltrate is superficial and rich in lymphocytes.

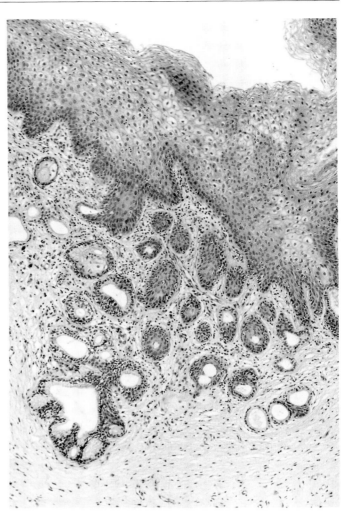

Figure 3.25. Vulvar vestibulitis with underlying minor vestibular glands. The epithelial surface is stratified squamous epithelium that is glycogen rich. Within the underlying tissue minor vestibular glands are present that are simple tubular glands with a mucous-secreting columnar epithelial lining. In some glands the columnar epithelium has been replaced by metaplastic squamous epithelium.

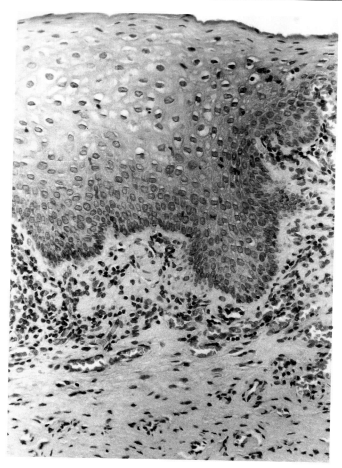

Figure 3.26. Vulvar vestibulitis. The glycogen-rich, nonkeratinized, squamous epithelium is similar to vaginal epithelium in women of reproductive age. There is a superficial subepithelial chronic inflammatory infiltrate that consists predominately of lymphocytes. Plasma cells are also present in approximately two-thirds of the cases.

Vitiligo

DEFINITION

Vitiligo is a lack of skin pigmentation secondary to absence of or diminished numbers of melanocytes.

GENERAL FEATURES

Vitiligo is thought to be an autosomal dominantly inherited disorder with variable penetrance. There is evidence of an autoimmune component to the condition. As many as one-third of patients may demonstrate thyroid dysfunction. Other associated conditions include Addison's disease, pernicious anemia, and diabetes mellitus.

CLINICAL PRESENTATION

Most patients with vulvar vitiligo will have no complaints and the hypopigmentation will be noted only if the patient observes the pigmentation disorder on self-examination or her sexual partner observes the depigmented skin. She may present with concerns about possibly infectious or neoplastic sources of depigmentation. Frequently, vitiligo will be present in other body sites in addition to the genitalia. These regions of depigmentation will have been long standing and the patient may be reassured that the vulvar condition is identical to the extragenital vitiligo. Vulvar vitiligo is frequently a symmetric process with sharply demarcated borders. The condition will be more apparent in dark-skinned patients than in light-skinned ones.

MICROSCOPIC FINDINGS

Vitiligo is rarely biopsied. No significant pathologic findings are evident; however, neither melanin pigment nor melanocytes are present.

ADDITIONAL STUDIES

Consideration should be given to an assay for thyroid function, given the frequent association between these vitiligo and thyroid dysfunction.

DIFFERENTIAL DIAGNOSIS

Vitiligo may be confused with lichen sclerosus because both conditions appear as pale vulvar skin. Vitiligo is a much more sharply demarcated condition. Whereas lichen sclerosus skin appears atrophic, patients with vitiligo have normal skin texture. Although patients with vitiligo occasionally may note pruritus, this is not a common complaint. Lichen sclerosus patients almost invariably complain of pruritus. Squamous cell hyperplasia may be another consideration, but the skin appears hyperkeratotic and pruritus is commonly noted.

CLINICAL BEHAVIOR AND TREATMENT

No therapy is needed or warranted for vitiligo involving the vulva. If the patient is overly concerned about the depigmented vulvar skin and requests an effort to improve or enhance pigmentation, a trial of moderate- to high-dose steroid creams or ointments may be attempted. If medium- to high-dose steroids are used, the intertriginous regions should be avoided. After a course of 1 to 2 months of daily applications, therapy may be tapered to a low-dose steroid, or discontinued for 1 to 2 months to allow recovery from the moderate- to high-dose steroid applications. It may take several months to see results from the steroid application. If no success is noted then the patient should be referred to a dermatologist for consideration of psoralen photochemotherapy. Other options include dermal tattooing and grafting.

Progressive Therapeutic Options

1. Reassurance that vitiligo is not a neoplastic process. Local cosmetics may be used to cover the hypopigmented skin if the patient perceives this to be cosmetically disfiguring.

2. For localized vitiligo of significant concern to the patient, topical medium- to high-dose steroid creams or ointments may be used daily for 4–8 weeks avoiding intertriginous zones. Therapy may be then tapered to a lower dose steroid or discontinued for several weeks to determine response and allow recovery from high-dose steroids.

3. Referral to dermatology for psoralen photochemotherapy or tattooing.

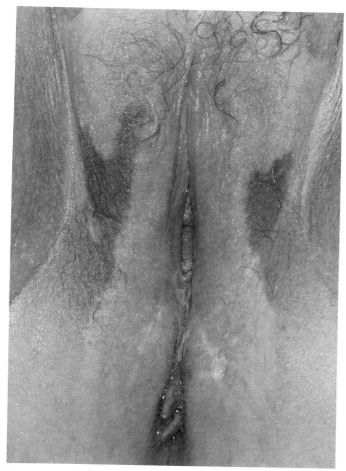

Figure 3.27. Hypopigmented symmetric pattern of vitiligo in a patient without symptoms.

4

PAPILLAE

PAPILLAE ALGORITHM

PAPILLA (Latin papula: pimple):
a nipple-shaped projection.

Location	*Presumed Diagnosis*
Vestibule	Squamous papillomatosis
	Condyloma acuminatum
	Fibroepithelial polyp

Figure 4.1. Papillae algorithm.

Squamous Vestibular Papillomatosis

DEFINITION

Squamous vestibular papillomatosis is the term used to describe small, usually multiple, papillary projections occurring within the vestibule exterior to the hymenal ring.

GENERAL FEATURES

These lesions may be seen frequently in both asymptomatic and symptomatic women. Their clinical relevance is controversial.

CLINICAL PRESENTATION

In a busy gynecologic practice, squamous vestibular papillomatosis may be seen frequently in asymptomatic women. Those patients who present with symptoms usually complain of pruritus or burning, especially associated with intercourse. Upon examination, small papillary projections will be noted, usually in a horseshoe-shaped distribution extending in a linear fashion down the medial aspect of the vestibule. Occasionally the papillae will extend throughout the medial aspect of the labia minora. There may be tenderness in this region, when touched with a cotton swab. Colposcopic examination after application of acetic acid may further highlight the papillae and occasionally demonstrate thickened white epithelium on the papillae, suggestive of human papillomavirus. There does not appear to be a causal relationship between human papillomavirus and the evolution of these papillary projections.

MICROSCOPIC FINDINGS

A vestibular papilloma is characterized by its origin from the vestibule, its relatively small size, ranging usually from 1 to 2 mm and rarely over 5 mm in length, and its epithelial surface, which is typically stratified squamous epithelium, glycogenated in women of reproductive age. On rare occasion, a thin keratin layer may be found. The fibrous core of the papilloma has a central vessel and loose connective stroma. This can be distinguished from condyloma accuminatum in that they do not exhibit keratinocyte mullinucleation, nuclear enlargement with typical koilocytosis, crowding of the basal and parabasal epithelial cells, accentuation of intercellular bridges, or a prominent keratin surface with or without parakeratosis. They are distinguished from fibroepithelial polyps by their size, location, and architecture.

CLINICAL BEHAVIOR AND TREATMENT

Symptomatic squamous vestibular papillomatosis may be treated in a variety of fashions. Any approach to therapy should take into consideration cost-effectiveness. Topical applications of trichloroacetic acid will often effect resolution of the papillae. Obviously this is painful and may require topical or local anesthesia. Topical 5% 5-fluorouracil (Efudex) may be applied once or twice daily for approximately 2 weeks. A chemical vulvitis is frequently seen in association with this topical use of 5-fluorouracil, and the patient may require topical anesthetics and should be forewarned of this possibility. The use of 5-fluorouracil should be avoided in pregnancy and not used in women of reproductive age when pregnancy is a concern. Cryotherapy and laser therapy also may result in resolution of the papillae. Patients should be forewarned that discomfort may persist after destruction of the papillae and vulvar vestibulitis may be associated and persist after destruction of the papillae. This should be discussed with the patient well in advance of therapeutic intervention. If the patient has symptoms of vestibulitis before the initiation of therapy for vestibular papillae, it is important to document and discuss this with the patient to preclude the perception that the vestibulitis symptoms developed as a result of local attempts to destroy the squamous papillomatosis.

Progressive Therapeutic Options

1. For symptomatic and possibly for human papillomavirus-associated asymptomatic squamous papillomatosis, apply topical trichloroacetic acid. Usually one application will be effective; however, a second application may be necessary in 2–3 weeks. Forewarn patient about discomfort and provide local anesthesia and analgesia as needed.
2. Topical application of 5% 5-fluorouracil once or twice daily for 2 weeks (forewarn of chemical vulvitis/vestibulitis). Pregnancy must be absolutely avoided with use of 5-fluorouracil.
3. Fine-tip cryotherapy or liquid nitrogen applications.
4. Laser ablation.

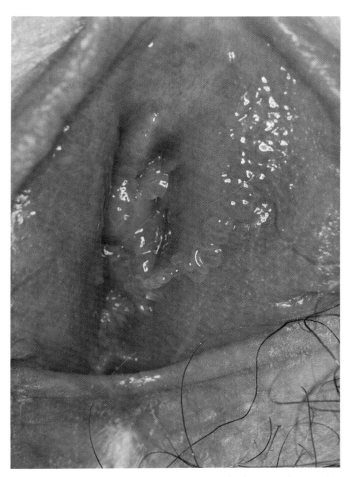

Figure 4.2. Patient with typical papillary projections consistent with squamous papillomatosis.

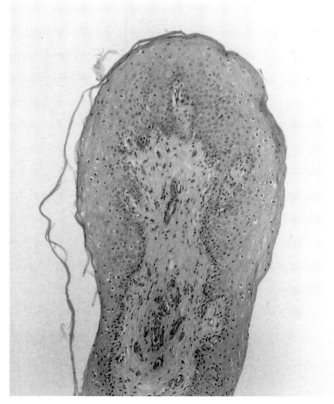

Figure 4.3. Vestibular papilloma. The surface-stratified squamous epithelium is glycogen rich. The fibrovascular stalk contains a central muscular vessel.

5

PAPULES

PAPULE ALGORITHM

PAPULE (Latin papula: pimple):
a small, discrete, solid elevation

Description	Presumed Diagnosis
Solitary	Compound nevus
	Dysplastic nevus
	Hairy cell nevus
	Intradermal nevus
	Pyogenic granuloma
	Seborrheic keratosis
Solitary (discharge)	Sinus tract
Multiple (red)	Angiokeratoma
Multiple (umbilicated)	Molluscum contagiosum

Figure 5.1. Papule algorithm.

Angiokeratoma

DEFINITION

Angiokeratomas are papular vascular lesions containing ectatic subepithelial dermal blood vessels that abut the basal epithelial layer.

GENERAL FEATURES

The etiology for these vascular lesions is unknown. Although they are frequently seen in vulvar clinics, the actual incidence in the population at large is unknown.

CLINICAL PRESENTATION

The patient with an angiokeratoma will usually be asymptomatic. The lesion will be noted on routine pelvic examination by the examining gynecologist. Rarely an angiokeratoma may ulcerate and bleed. Upon examining the asymptomatic patient with an angiokeratoma, a small 2–5-mm papular lesion will be noted on the vulva. Unless it has been irritated, it will not be tender. Color ranges from a dark red to purplish hue. Multiple angiokeratomas may be noted in patients with Fabry's disease. Fabry's disease is an X-linked recessive disease associated with a deficiency of α-galactosidase A, resulting in deposition of glycosphingolipids throughout a number of body tissues. The disease usually affects men and may be fatal in the fourth and fifth decades of life. The interesting dermatologic observation is the occurrence of multiple angiokeratomas on the skin. Very rarely the disease may be noted in women in the heterozygous state. Heterozygous women usually do not have a severe form of the disease; however, they may have renal involvement resulting in proteinuria, corneal involvement resulting in corneal opacities, neurologic involvement resulting in paresthesias, and dermatologic involvement resulting in angiokeratomas.

MICROSCOPIC FINDINGS

Angiokeratomas are considered variants of hemangiomas. They are characterized by prominent endothelial-lined, blood-filled vascular channels immediately beneath the basement membrane of the overlying epithelium and separated by the rete ridges of the epithelium. These ridges form epithelial cords, which separate the vascular channels, resulting in a multilocular, lobulated appearance to the angiokeratoma. The overlying epithelium usually has some degree of acanthosis and papillomatosis, as well as hyperkeratosis. A mild chronic inflammatory infiltrate may be seen in the dermis beneath the vascular channels.

ADJUNCTIVE STUDIES

A patient with multiple angiokeratomas on the vulva should receive consideration for screening for Fabry's disease. This is accomplished by obtaining a white blood cell α-galactosidase activity. If the α-galactosidase activity is subnormal, then the patient should be counseled concerning her heterozygous state for Fabry's disease and family members should be screened appropriately. Pregnant carriers of the disease may choose to undergo amniocentesis or chorionic villi sampling to assess for potential fetal involvement with this significant disease.

CLINICAL BEHAVIOR AND TREATMENT

Treatment for angiokeratomas is warranted in symptomatic patients. Otherwise they may be observed without intervention. The diagnosis should be confirmed before ablative procedures are done because atypical nevi may also present as papular hyperpigmented lesions on the vulva. Excision is easily performed in the clinical setting. It is usually not necessary to take these patients to the operating room; however, multiple lesions requiring numerous incisions or laser ablation may require anesthesia in the operating room. There is a tendency for angiokeratomas to recur and the patient should be forewarned of this. As they recur and become symptomatic, they may be removed individually in the office. Excisions do not need to be deep because these dermal vessels are not deeply seated. Bleeding is usually minimal with their removal. Skin may be left to heal by secondary intention with small lesions, or may be approximated with a single stitch of appropriate suture material after excising larger lesions.

Progressive Therapeutic Options

1. After biopsy confirms the diagnosis, asymptomatic lesions may be followed.
2. Symptomatic lesions may be excised. Multiple lesions may be treated with cryotherapy or with laser ablation.

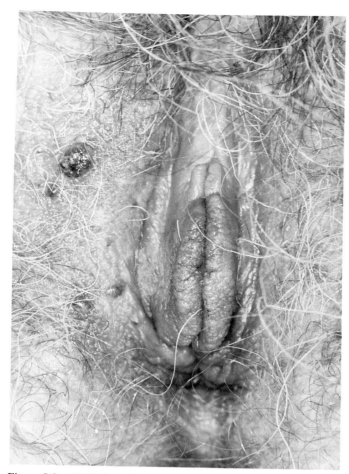

Figure 5.2. Multiple angiokeratomas in a woman with white blood cell alpha-galactosidase of 36 nM/hr/mg (normal = 50–80). Diagnosis of Fabry's disease was made and lesions were ablated with a laser.

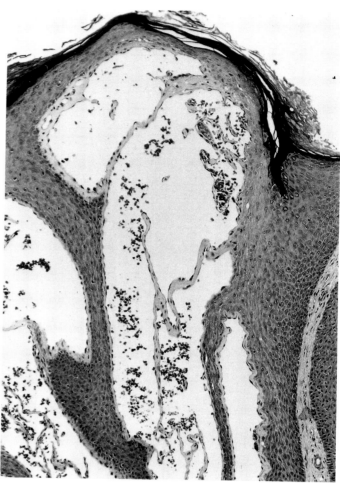

Figure 5.3. Angiokeratoma. Prominent dilated, blood-filled vessels are present immediately beneath the epithelium, and abut the epithelium. The overlying epithelium has markedly elongated rete ridges that are immediately adjacent to the dilated vascular channels.

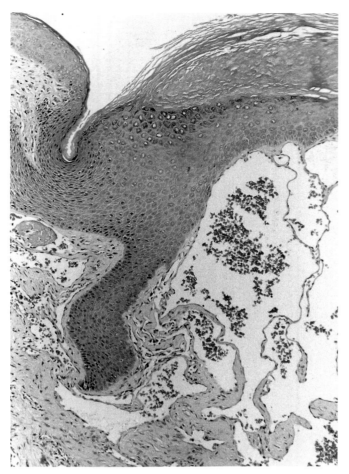

Figure 5.4. Angiokeratoma. The immediate proximity of the vascular endothelium to the overlying epithelium is evident.

Molluscum Contagiosum

DEFINITION

Molluscum contagiosum is a pox virus infection that results in formation of papular, centrally umbilicated skin lesions.

GENERAL FEATURES

Historically the disease has been common in children, but is increasingly seen in vulvar clinic patients and immunosuppressed patients.

CLINICAL PRESENTATION

Many patients with molluscum contagiosum will be unaware of the vulvar lesions that have resulted from sexual contact or autoinoculation from sites distant from the vulva. The symptomatic patient will present for evaluation of small papular lesions noted upon self-examination. Unless the lesions have been irritated and secondarily infected, they are usually asymptomatic. The patient will express concerns that she has a venereal disease such as condyloma acuminatum and will request evaluation and therapy. Upon examination the classic, centrally umbilicated papular lesion will be noted. The lesion may be solitary but more frequently occurs in clusters. Rarely a papule may be quite large and pedunculated without central umbilication.

The diagnosis is suspected immediately upon observation of the classic lesion or lesions. Confirmation of the diagnosis is made by histologic examination of an excised papule but usually this will not be required. Pressure upon the outer edges of the papule will result in extravasation of the central core, which is characteristic of molluscum contagiosum. Occasionally it will be necessary to obtain a specimen for histologic diagnosis. This will be the case with the large pedunculated papule, which may be confused with an acrochordon or nevus.

MICROSCOPIC FINDINGS

The lesions of molluscum contagiosum usually are not biopsied. Cytologic smears of the extruded contents of a molluscum lesion demonstrate epithelial cells with characteristic intracytoplasmic inclusions (molluscum bodies). The cytoplasmic inclusion is usually eosinophilic, but may be basophilic in older lesions. The virus-rich inclusions are released with death of the epithelial cell.

Cross-section of the lesion, at right angles to the epithelium and through the central surface dimple,

demonstrates the lesion to be entirely intraepithelial with prominent acanthosis about the central core. The core contains the epithelial cells containing molluscum bodies. The core containing infected, degenerated keratinocytes communicates with the surface at the dimpled epithelium. An inflammatory cell infiltrate is present within the superficial dermis, which usually extends perivascularly. Endothelial cell proliferation is evident in these involved areas.

Electron microscopy demonstrates the brick-shaped virus, which measures 300 mm ×20 mm and has a DNA core with a two-layered protein coat.

ADJUNCTIVE STUDIES

Immunosuppressed patients may be at higher risk for acquiring this viral infection; therefore, patients with molluscum contagiosum should be considered candidates for testing for the human immunodeficiency virus.

CLINICAL BEHAVIOR AND TREATMENT

Traditionally, molluscum contagiosum has been allowed to regress in young children without intervention. Lesions will frequently resolve, although the process may take several months. Most likely this approach has been secondary to a reluctance to perform painful evacuation of the papules in small children. Adults with molluscum contagiosum will be reluctant to follow a program of observation. As the name implies, the lesions are contagious. They are managed easily by evacuation. The lesions may be curetted with either a small curette or the end of a needle (18-gauge). Local anesthesia is not typically required. Bleeding from the base of the lesion may be easily controlled with Monsel's solution or silver nitrate. Chemical destruction of papules may be accomplished with applications of trichloroacetic acid at 1- to 2-week intervals. The patient should be forewarned of the potential for development for scarring and hyperpigmentation after evacuation and chemical cautery. Alternatively, lesions may be destroyed with cryotherapy or liquid nitrogen application. Very fine applicator tips are required to minimize lateral tissue destruction. Electrodesiccation is also an alternative but this will be painful. Laser therapy may be used but extensive scarring may result, with a less-than-optimal cosmetic result. Large, pedunculated, atypical molluscum contagiosum lesions will require sharp excision under local anesthesia for diagnostic purposes and therapeutic success.

Progressive Therapeutic Options

1. Evacuation by curettage and placement of chemical cauterizing agents to the base of the papule (silver nitrate or Monsel's solution).
2. Trichloroacetic acid application at 1- to 2-week intervals.
3. Cryotherapy or liquid nitrogen application to the papule with fine-tipped applicators.
4. Laser therapy (forewarning patient of potential for scar formation).
5. Excision of large lesions for diagnosis and therapy.

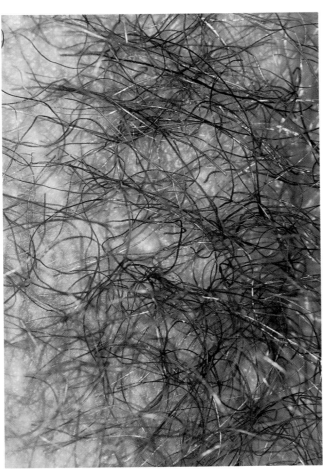

Figure 5.5. Typical papular lesion noted with molluscum contagiosum infection.

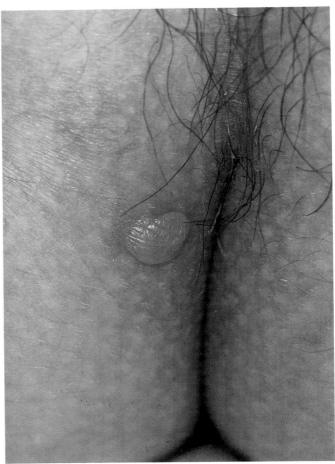

Figure 5.6. Atypical broad-based lesion with biopsy-confirmed diagnosis of molluscum contagiosum.

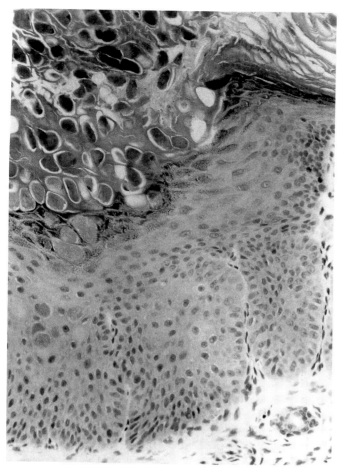

Figure 5.7. Molluscum contagiosum. This is the cup-like edge of the papule, where the epithelium is thickened and the overlying keratin ''plug'' contains many keratinocytes that have prominent, virus-rich cytoplasmic inclusions (molluscum bodies).

Nevi

DEFINITION

A skin tumor formed by clusters of neural crest-derived benign nevus cells within the dermis and epidermis.

GENERAL FEATURES

Nevi are found in the vast majority of the population but are not common on the vulvar skin.

CLINICAL PRESENTATION

Nevi observed at birth are termed congenital nevi. Large congenital nevi have a higher incidence of malignant transformation during the life-span of the person. Most nevi are not present at birth but develop over the ensuing years, frequently during adolescence. Sun-exposed areas of the body have a higher incidence of nevi. Most nevi will originate as junctional or flat nevi with minimal elevation above the surface skin. Contour is smooth and regular and the margins are well demarcated. Color is uniformly a shade of brown (ranging from tan to dark brown or black). The junctional nevus has nevus cells at the epidermal-dermal junction. As the nevus ages the nevus cells will migrate into the upper dermis; elevation of the overlying epithelium results in formation of a papular lesion. As with the junctional nevus, this compound nevus is demarcated with regular borders and the color is uniform. As this lesion ages, nevus cells will become predominantly located in the dermis, forming an intradermal nevus. The intradermal nevus may appear pedunculated or polypoid.

Patients with vulvar nevi will most frequently complain of symptoms associated with compound and intradermal nevi. These nevi are readily palpated and may become irritated. The junctional nevus is rarely observed by the patient unless she visualizes it during self-examination. More commonly the junctional nevus is observed by an examining physician during routine examination. Concern with the potential for a melanoma will usually prompt diagnostic evaluation.

The diagnosis of nevus is easily suspected upon visual examination. The junctional nevus will be flat or slightly elevated, the compound nevus will be more papular, and the intradermal nevus may be papular, polypoid, or pedunculated. Because melanomas may also appear as slightly elevated, papular, or polypoid, concern always exists that one is dealing with a melanoma of the vulva. Melanomas will be irregular in contour with poorly defined margins. There will be significant variations in color throughout the body of the melanoma. These physical characteristics will prompt a biopsy or excisional biopsy to rule out melanoma. Because uncertainty often exists with clinical diagnosis, most hyperpigmented lesions of the vulva should be excised or biopsied for histologic confirmation of diagnosis. To augment the clinician's visual inspection, the colposcope may be used to magnify a nevus to define the character of the lesion further. Lentigo simplex is a common finding in older patients and is typically a flat or slightly papular hyperpigmented lesion. The borders are somewhat irregular. A patient with lentigo simplex may have numerous lentigines on the vulva, especially within the vestibule. It may be difficult to differentiate lentigo simplex from a junctional nevus based on visual inspection. Larger areas of pigmentation without epithelial changes that are confluent are termed *melanosis* and are histologically indistinguishable from lentigo simplex. When dealing with a large area of hyperpigmented skin, a diagnostic biopsy rather than an excisional biopsy may be more appropriate. This diagnostic biopsy should be through the thickest and darkest region of the lesion and should be transdermal to the subcuticular adipose tissue. A wedge section can then be submitted for pathologic confirmation of diagnosis. Smaller lesions may be totally excised, provided adequate margins are maintained.

MICROSCOPIC FINDINGS

Nevi are composed of nevomelanocytic cells, which are slightly larger than melanocytes and have round to oval nuclei and little cytoplasm. They do not have dendrites nor do they exhibit intercellular bridges. The cytoplasm may contain melanin; however, most nevi have a relatively clear cytoplasm.

Vulvar nevi can be classified according to the location of the nevomelanocytic cells.

Junctional nevi are composed of nevomelanocytes, which are clustered at the epidermal-dermal junction, forming a "nest of cells." Pure junctional nevi are rare on the vulva and are considered the earliest form of nevus development. As nevi mature, the epidermal basement membrane regresses about the nevus and dermal collagen elastic fibers and reticulum surround the nevus, which initially results in the nevus being within the dermis as well as epithelium. Such nevi are classified as compound nevi. More mature nevi will be completely within the dermis, and these are classified as intradermal.

Most nevi excised from the vulva are compound or intradermal.

ATYPICAL VULVAR NEVI

A small percent of vulvar nevi have mild cellular atypia in the junctional component and they have been referred to as atypical vulvar nevi. They are usually 4 cm or less in diameter and are compound nevi. These lesions are typically symmetrical on cross-section, have maturation of the nevomelanocytes in the dermis, have no significant pagetoid spread, and lack mitosis in the nevomelanocytic component. They are not associated with the dysplastic nevus syndrome; however, the syndrome should be considered when such nevi are identified. The major differential is to distinguish such atypical compound nevi from malignant melanoma.

CLINICAL BEHAVIOR AND TREATMENT

The vast majority of nevi require no therapy; however, concern regarding the potential for malignancy results in excision of most vulvar nevi. Obviously symptomatic nevi with irritation and bleeding should be excised for therapy and diagnosis. The elderly patient who is noted to have a polypoid lesion on the vulva which has been present for many years without change most likely has either an intradermal nevus or acrochordon, which may be followed without excision. It is highly unlikely that such a lesion would undergo malignant degeneration in an elderly woman who has noted no change over a number of years. At the other end of the age spectrum is the adolescent female noted to have a hyperpigmented lesion on the vulva. Concern exists that a large junctional nevus at this age may evolve into a melanoma during the patient's life span. When dealing with hyperpigmented elevated papular or pedunculated lesions of the vulva, the preferred approach is therapeutic and diagnostic excision. Vulvar melanosis may be biopsied and followed after histology confirms a benign diagnosis. When excising an elevated or suspicious hyperpigmented vulvar lesion, the entire lesion should be removed and the excision should extend to the subcutaneous fat with adequate margins obtained for histologic clearance.

Progressive Therapeutic Option

1. Excisional biopsy for histologic diagnosis and therapeutic removal of vulvar hyperpigmented lesions.

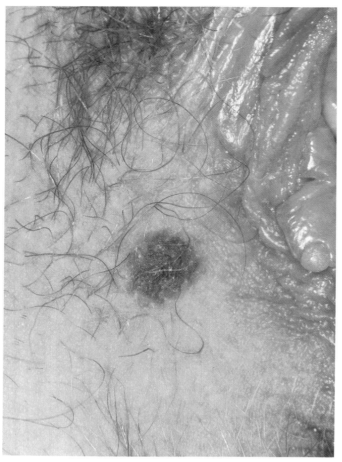

Figure 5.8. Irregular, variegated nevus in 20-year-old woman. Lesion was excised and histology was consistent with compound nevus.

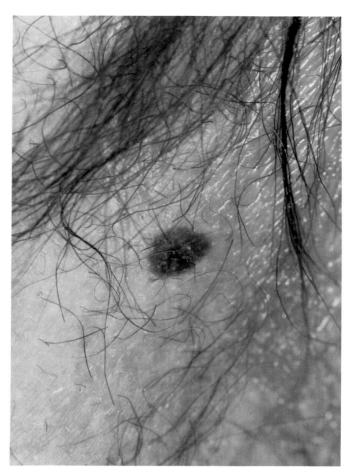

Figure 5.9. Melanotic, homogenous nevus believed clinically to be a compound nevus. Histology was consistent with an intradermal nevus.

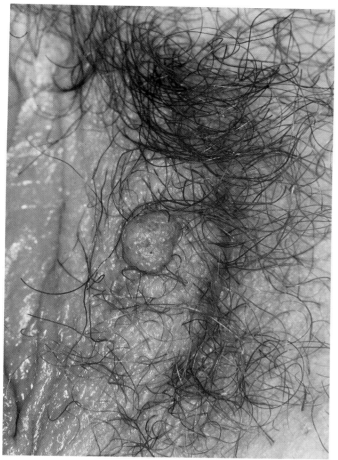

Figure 5.10. Elevated, homogenous nevus suggestive of intradermal nevus; however, histologic diagnosis was compound nevus.

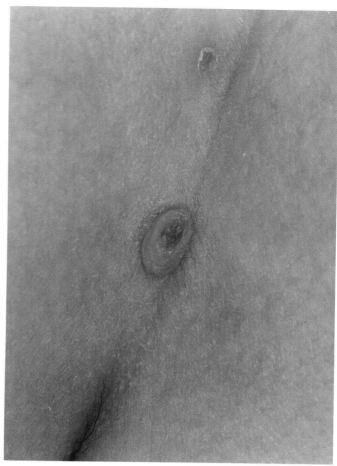

Figure 5.11. Congenital intradermal hairy nevus in a 35-year-old patient.

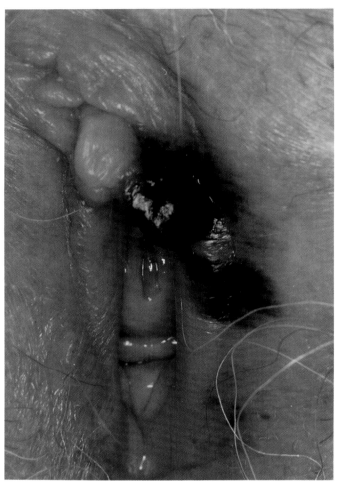

Figure 5.12. Malignant melanoma. Patient also had multiple ulcerative lesions on the soles of her feet. Note the dark hue and irregular borders. (Photo courtesy of F. W. McLean, M.D.)

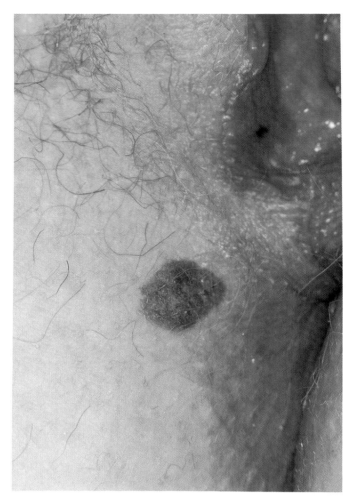

Figure 5.13. Atypical vulvar nevus in an adolescent patient.

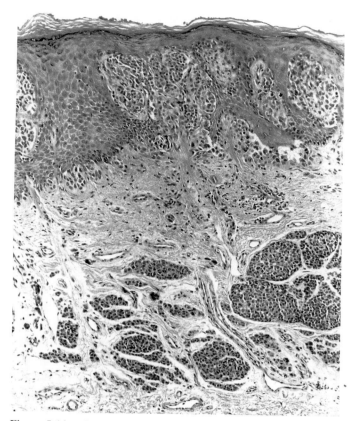

Figure 5.14. Compound vulvar nevus with atypia. The overlying epithelium is slightly thinned with prominent rete ridges. Nests of nevomelanocytic cells are within the epidermal-dermal junction and nearly fill the papillary dermis. In the deeper dermis, well-defined nests of mature nevomelanocytic cells are identified.

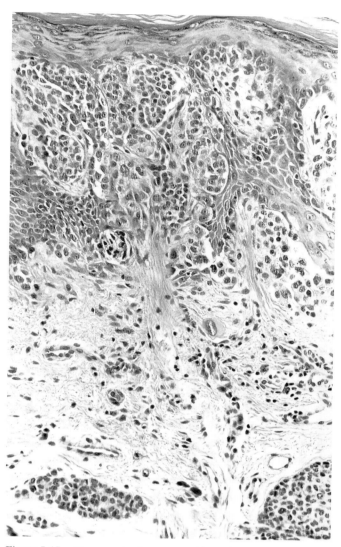

Figure 5.15. Compound vulvar nevus with atypia. A high magnification of the junctional area demonstrates the mild atypia of the junctional nevomelanocytic cells and the lack of pagetoid spread of these cells into the epithelium.

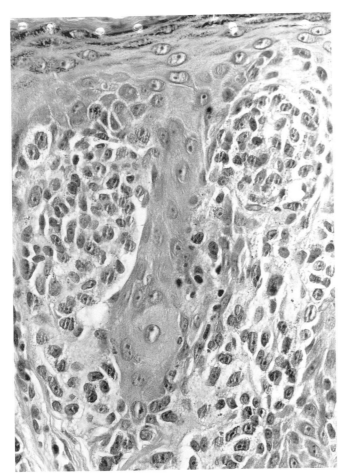

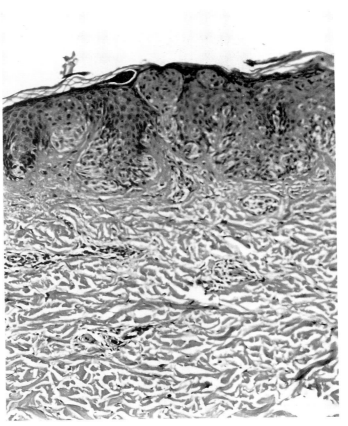

Figure 5.16. Compound vulvar nevus with atypia. A higher magnification of the adjacent field illustrates the nests of nevomelanocytic cells within the junctional area of the epithelium. Pagetoid intraepithelial spread within the epidermis is not identified. The deeper nests of nevus cells are small, have a relatively uniform shape, and are mature in appearance compared with those cells in the junctional area (see Fig. 5.15).

Figure 5.17. Superficial spreading malignant melanoma. Nests of melanocytes fill the papillary dermis and obscure the epithelial dermal junction. The nests extend into the upper epidermis. Pagetoid spread of the melanocytes is evident within the epithelium.

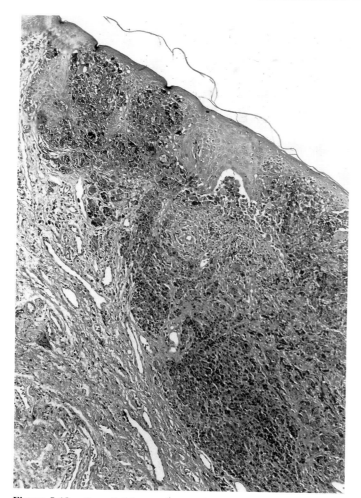

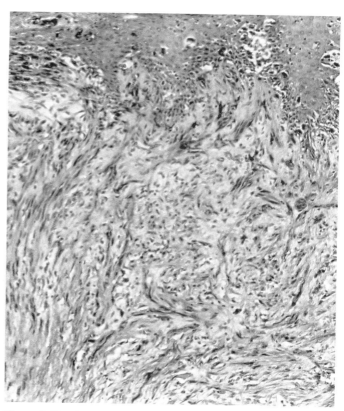

Figure 5.19. Spindle-cell melanoma. Most of the tumor cells are elongated and spindle shaped. Melanin is not present. The tumor involves the overlying epithelium.

Figure 5.18. Superficial spreading malignant melanoma with vertical (invasive) growth. The superficial spreading component is present adjacent to the invasive melanoma. Melanin pigment is present in the superficial spreading and invasive components. The tumor has eroded the overlying epithelium.

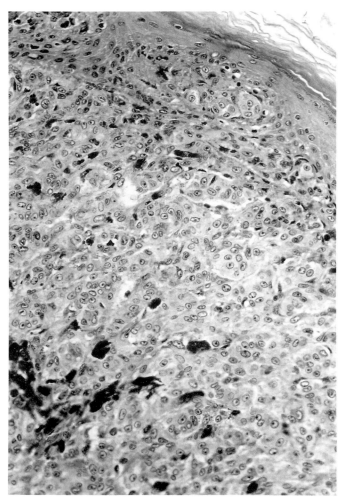

Figure 5.20. Nodular malignant melanoma. This tumor had no superficial spreading component. The tumor involves the epithelium and deeply
infiltrates the dermis. The tumor cells are large and pleomorphic, with
vesicular nuclear chromatin and prominent nucleoli. Some of the melanoma cells contain melanin.

Pyogenic Granuloma (Lobular Capillary Hemangioma, Granuloma Telangiectaticum)

DEFINITION

A highly vascular papule usually developing at a site of previous injury.

GENERAL FEATURES

Pyogenic granuloma, contrary to its implication, probably has no association with an infectious origin. The lesion is most commonly seen in areas of recent trauma, usually on the extremities and face. It has a propensity to occur in children. It is seen during pregnancy as the granuloma gravidarum involving the oral mucosa (specifically the gums).

CLINICAL PRESENTATION

The patient will present with a rapidly developing papular lesion on the vulva that may have bled. On examination, a papule will be noted. The color may be bright red or bluish-black. Older lesions may be ulcerated and crusted. The lesion is not tender upon examination but may bleed easily when touched. Occasionally there may be satellite lesions surrounding a larger central lesion.

MICROSCOPIC FEATURES

Pyogenic granuloma is a benign vascular neoplasm that is characterized microscopically by epithelial ulceration with underlying prominent dermal vascularity, resembling granulation tissue, with edema and inflammation. The ulcer has a surrounding collarete that is composed of a thickened and acanthotic epidermis. Beneath the ulcer surface a central vascular lobule is present that consists of a core of clustered vessels with surrounding smaller vessels that have prominent endothelial cells. The vessels of the vascular lobule usually do not contain red blood cells and are surrounded by edematous fibrous tissue that usually contains some chronic inflammatory cells.

DIFFERENTIAL DIAGNOSIS

The appearance of a rapidly growing lesion in a region of prior injury or in a region exposed to injury should raise the suspicion of pyogenic granuloma. Often, however, patients will have no history of trauma. The differential diagnosis should include nevi, malignant melanoma, molluscum contagiosum, and angiokeratoma. Confirmation of diagnosis can be obtained only by excisional biopsy.

CLINICAL BEHAVIOR AND TREATMENT

It is rare for a pyogenic granuloma to recede spontaneously. The lesion will persist and continue to bleed until excised. Full excision is required to remove all proliferating capillaries. Unless the entire lesion is removed it will recur. Multiple recurrent lesions may arrange themselves as a rosette around the previously excised central lesion. Although cryocautery may be an alternative, transdermal destruction of the capillary proliferation is not ensured and excision is the preferred mode of management. Children presenting with vulvar pyogenic granulomas should be considered at risk for sexual abuse and an appropriate history and evaluation should be obtained.

Progressive Therapeutic Option

1. Transdermal excision of lesion and suture approximation of wound. Specimen should be submitted to pathology laboratory for confirmation of diagnosis.

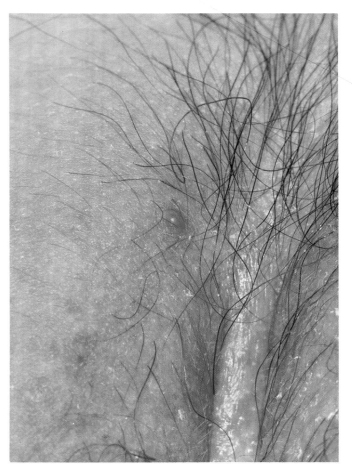

Figure 5.21. Pyogenic granuloma recurring near the sulcus between the right labium majus and right labium minus in a young girl. The early papule is neither ulcerated nor is it friable. It may be confused easily with molluscum contagiosum, although there is no central umbilication.

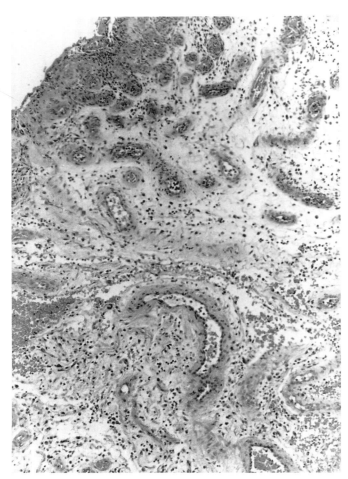

Figure 5.22. Pyogenic granuloma. This is epithelial ulceration with associated acute and chronic inflammation. Prominent small vessels are present in the superficial ulcer, as seen in granulation tissue. A central larger vessel is usually present in the adjacent deeper dermis. The adjacent epithelium is hyperplastic.

Seborrheic Keratosis

DEFINITION

A seborrheic keratosis is a benign papular intraepithelial lesion with hyperkeratosis, keratin horn cysts, acanthosis, and papillomatosis within the epidermis.

GENERAL FEATURES

Seborrheic keratoses are frequently seen in older persons but are relatively rare on the vulva. More often they are seen on the face and trunk. They are not considered premalignant. The sudden appearance and rapid increase in size and number of seborrheic keratoses may be associated with internal malignancy, specifically of the gastrointestinal tract (the sign of Leser-Trélat).

CLINICAL PRESENTATION

A vulvar seborrheic keratosis may be discovered by the patient on self examination. The lesion will be slightly elevated above the skin, will be well demarcated, and usually will be pigmented. The surface may appear waxy, hence the term seborrheic. The lesion may appear to have been pasted on the skin. Usually there will be no associated symptoms unless the lesion is being irritated by undergarments. The patient may be concerned that the lesion is premalignant or malignant. Perhaps more frequently the lesions are noted by an examining gynecologist on routine examination, and when questioned the patient will note that the lesion has been present for a number of years without change. It is extremely unusual to find multiple seborrheic keratoses on the vulva.

MICROSCOPIC FEATURES

The histologic findings include prominent acanthosis and papillomatosis with hyperkeratosis with keratin horn cysts. A useful diagnostic feature is the finding, on low-power examination, that the deepest edges of the acanthotic rete ridges lie above a straight line drawn between the bilaterally adjacent normal epithelial deep dermal papillae. Horney keratinous cysts within the epithelium are surrounded by basalar and mature keratinocytes. Melanin pigment may be present in basal keratinocytes. This pigmentation can be highly variable and accounts for the dark color of some seborrheic keratoses.

ADJUNCTIVE STUDIES

Evaluation for internal malignancy would only be indicated if, as noted above, there had been a sudden appearance of or sudden increase in the number and size of seborrheic keratoses. The discovery of an isolated seborrheic keratosis that has been stable for years is not an indication to perform radiologic and endoscopic evaluations of the gastrointestinal tract to rule out malignancy.

DIFFERENTIAL DIAGNOSIS

A seborrheic keratosis is classic in appearance; however, other conditions may simulate this process. Included in the differential diagnosis would be condyloma acuminatum, vulvar intraepithelial neoplasia, basal cell carcinoma, compound nevus, intradermal nevus, and melanoma.

CLINICAL BEHAVIOR AND TREATMENT

Seborrheic keratosis is a benign condition. Removal is indicated when the diagnosis is uncertain or when the condition is symptomatic. Because the process involves only the epidermis, the classic seborrheic keratosis may be curetted after accomplishing local anesthesia. Small lesions also may be treated with cryotherapy. When uncertainty exists concerning the diagnosis and the specimen is being removed for histologic confirmation, transcutaneous excisional biopsy is preferred to provide the pathologist with an appropriately representative segment of skin to rule out such premalignant conditions as intraepithelial neoplasia and such malignant lesions as melanoma. Large lesions of uncertain histology may be approached with a representative biopsy through the thickest region, and final disposition will be based upon pathologic review. If pathology confirms a seborrheic keratosis, then the patient may return for a sharp curettage of the lesion.

Progressive Therapeutic Options

1. Excisional biopsy of small lesions will confirm the diagnosis and remove a symptomatic keratosis.
2. Larger lesions may be biopsied and if the diagnosis is confirmed, the patient may return for sharp curettage or excision under local anesthesia.

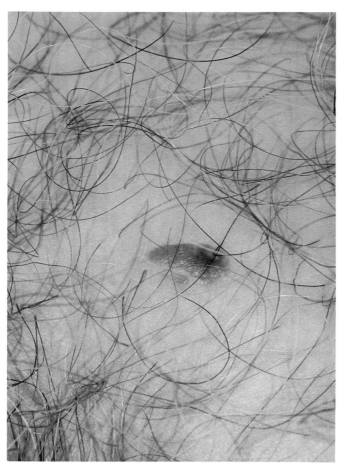

Figure 5.23. Typical waxy surface of biopsy-confirmed vulvar seborrheic keratosis.

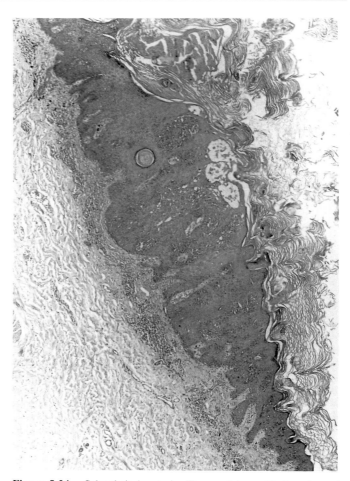

Figure 5.24. Seborrheic keratosis. The overlying epithelium is markedly acanthotic with hyperkeratosis and an intraepithelial keratin "pearl." Note that the entire lesion is above a line drawn from the epithelial dermal junction of the adjacent epithelium.

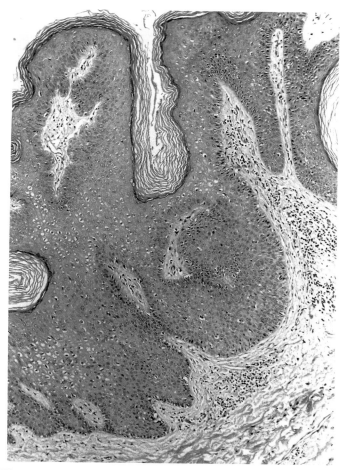

Figure 5.25. Seborrheic keratosis. The epithelium is thickened and hyperkeratotic; however, no significant cytoatypia is present. A superficial chronic inflammatory infiltrate is present within the superficial dermis.

Sinus Tract (Fistula-in-Ano)

DEFINITION

A sinus tract or fistula is an epithelialized tract observed in association with chronic inflammatory or infectious disease processes that communicates with a visceral organ, abscess cavity, or an adjacent epithelial surface.

GENERAL FEATURES

The sinus tract has an external, or secondary, opening and an internal, or primary, site of infection or inflammation, often with an opening in the bowel lumen. If this opening is in the anus near the dentate line, the designation *fistula-in-ano* is used. A sinus tract may be observed as a consequence of a crypt abscess at the dentate line in the anus or as a consequence of chronic inflammatory bowel disease such as Crohn's disease. A tract may occur as a consequence of such chronic inflammatory dermatologic conditions as hidradenitis suppurativa, where the sinus tract opens to the epithelial surface.

CLINICAL PRESENTATION

The patient with a perianal sinus tract or fistula will usually present complaining of drainage of a serous or mucopurulent discharge that soils the underwear. Rarely there may be a history of an antecedent perianal or perirectal abscess. The tract will have been present for weeks to months before the patient presents. On examination a raised area of apparent granulation tissue will be observed in the perianal region. On examination there will be extravasation of a mucopurulent or serous fluid from the external opening of the sinus tract. There may be mild tenderness present. The most common presentation will be that of a single sinus tract, usually anterior to a line drawn across the midsection of the anus, separating the anus into an anterior and posterior segment.

The diagnosis is confirmed by inserting a small lacrimal probe into the canal of the sinus tract. Gentle pressure is used to determine the course of the tract. Undue pressure will result in creation of a false tract and will not be helpful in determining where the primary, or internal, opening of the sinus originates. The examination is best accomplished with the examining physician's index finger in the anus while gently inserting the lacrimal probe through the external, or secondary, opening. Sinus tracts, which are anterior to an imaginary line drawn through the midportion of the anus, almost invari-

ably originate anteriorly and directly from the anal canal. Sinus tracts noted posterior to the line will frequently curve and enter the posterior midline of the anal canal (Goodsall's rule). Sinus tracts that are extremely lateral to the anus may course in any direction and may enter the bowel lumen significantly cephalad to the dentate line or may curve posteriorally and enter the posterior anal canal. Radiologic studies of these laterally placed lesions, which apparently enter high in the bowel lumen, should be accomplished to establish the site of the primary opening. Medial tracts can be evaluated in the office with a lacrimal probe to determine the primary origin in many instances. The primary origin of the tract unfortunately, is often too small to be determined with a lacrimal probe. Sterile milk may be injected into the tract's external opening, while visualizing the anal canal with an anal speculum in place. If the internal opening remains elusive, radiographic studies (sinogram) should be obtained to define the course of the lesion and the location of the internal opening.

MICROSCOPIC FINDINGS

Excised sinus tracts typically are associated with severe acute and chronic inflammation. The tract may or may not have an epithelial lining; however, near the squamous epithelial surface, some squamous epithelial cells can be found lining the tract. If the sinus tract is secondary to Crohn's disease, granulomas may be evident (see Crohn's disease). Giant cells are not characteristic. If foreign body giant cells are found, suture material or other foreign material may be present. Polarization of the tissue, employing polarizing lenses, is of value to identify polarizable foreign material. Histochemical stains for fungi and bacteria, including acid-fast bacteria, are of value for completeness, although rarely reveal organisms within the tissue.

DIFFERENTIAL DIAGNOSIS

The differential diagnosis of perianal and vulvar sinus tracts is limited. For patients with multiple lesions or for patients with sinus tracts originating high in the bowel lumen, inflammatory bowel disease should be considered. Endoscopic and radiographic studies of the bowel would be warranted in such patients.

Hidradenitis suppurativa does not involve the bowel lumen. Sinus tracts will be directed in a subcutaneous fashion, often deep into the fat but will not communicate with the bowel or vaginal opening.

Often there will also be involvement of the axillary regions with this inflammatory disease. Lymphogranuloma venereum will present in advanced stages as an anogenital syndrome with sinus tracts or fistulae involving the bowel. Marked edema of the vulva may be observed. Appropriate chlamydial serology should be obtained to exclude the possibility of this process.

CLINICAL BEHAVIOR AND TREATMENT

The treatment of an uncomplicated sinus tract is surgical. Successful surgical treatment requires excision of the inciting crypt or internal, primary opening. A primary opening often will be too small to be discerned and every effort should be made to excise what appears to be the primary source of the tract at the dentate line. A lacrimal probe may be placed in the sinus tract. The skin, muscle, and anal mucosa overlying the tract may be incised down to the lacrimal probe with healing by secondary intention. Alternatively, the tract may be excised, although this is often difficult, especially with a small sinus tract. If the effort to excise the tract is unsuccessful, curettage may be accomplished. Presence of an obviously infected sinus tract should prompt the operating surgeon to pursue a more conservative approach of unroofing the tract and allowing healing by secondary intention rather than closing the area primarily. The patient must be warned that recurrence is possible, especially if the primary site or

internal opening is too small for clinical detection. Sinus tracts that open posteriorly require more extensive surgery and dissection than those that open anteriorly. Surgery for perianal sinus tracts carries the risk of anal incontinence, which may require corrective surgery at a future date. Lesions originating high in the bowel lumen cephalad to the anal canal pose particular operative risks and cannot be approached as unroofing procedures. Such fistulae may require diverting procedures and are usually a consequence of inflammatory bowel disease. All efforts should be made to manage these patients nonsurgically.

Progressive Therapeutic Options

1. Appropriate presurgical evaluation to define the internal origin of the sinus tract and rule out inflammatory bowel disease, lymphogranuloma venereum, and hidradenitis suppurativa.
2. Surgical unroofing of the *superficial* sinus tract and excision of the primary opening or inciting inflamed crypt. The patient should be forewarned of the risk of anal incontinence developing from an unroofing procedure.
3. Excision of the *deeper* uninfected sinus tract with primary closure of all tissue planes, using appropriate antibiotic prophylaxis. The patient should be forewarned of the risk of recurrence and the risk of anal incontinence.

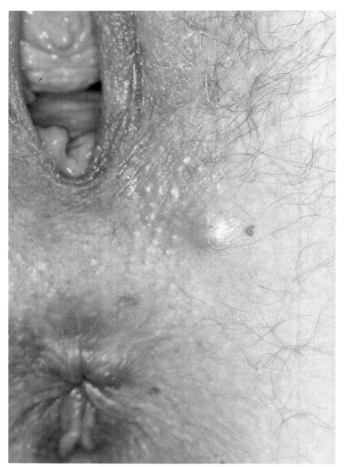

Figure 5.26. Typical solitary sinus tract. Tract was defined with methylene blue and excised to bowel wall but recurred within 6 months.

6

PLAQUES

PLAQUE ALGORITHM

PLAQUE (French plaquier: to plate): a flat, elevated lesion that may be formed by coalescing papules.

Color	Presumed Diagnosis
Red	Candidiasis
	Eczema
	Lichen simplex
	Paget's disease
	Plasma cell vulvitis
	Psoriasis
	Seborrhea
White/acetowhite	VIN
	Condyloma acuminatum
Hyperpigmented (dark)	VIN
	Nevi
	Melanoma

Figure 6.1. Plaque algorithm.

Candidiasis

DEFINITION

Candidiasis is a fungal infection most commonly caused by *Candida albicans*.

GENERAL FEATURES

Vulvar candidiasis is a fairly common external manifestation of a vaginal infection with *Candida*. Rarely does one see vulvar candidiasis without concomitant vaginal candidiasis. Candidiasis is often seen in patients who have altered immune systems, such as is noted in persons infected with the human immunodeficiency virus (HIV). Diabetic patients will have frequent bouts of candidiasis especially if the diabetes is under poor control. Candidiasis develops frequently after taking antibiotic therapy for extragenital infections such as pharyngitis, otis, and cystitis. Antibiotic therapy will alter the normal flora of the vagina and allow overgrowth of *Candida* species, resulting in vaginitis and vulvitis.

CLINICAL PRESENTATION

Patients with vulvar candidiasis most commonly will present with a complaint of an intense vulvar pruritus. There may also be an associated vaginal discharge. The vulva will be intensely erythematous and will often demonstrate a white adherent film. The medical history may not contain a history of diabetes. Because vulvar candidiasis may be the initial manifestation of occult diabetes mellitus, consideration should be given to obtaining a blood glucose level on patients with intense vulvar candidiasis or recurrent vulvar candidiasis. A patient who gives a recent history of antibiotic usage with resultant candidiasis does not routinely need a blood glucose assay. Nor would it be imperative to obtain HIV serostatus on such a patient. However, if no risk factors are noted for the development of recurrent candidiasis and the blood glucose studies are within normal limits, consideration should be given to obtaining an HIV assay after appropriate counseling.

MICROSCOPIC FINDINGS

The key histologic feature of candidiasis is the finding of acute inflammatory cells within the epithelium, with the identification of the fungal hyphae on silver fungus or periodic acid-Schiff stain. The epithelium may be acanthotic and hyperkeratotic, and the fungal organisms are found in the keratin layer. Superficial epithelial erosion with mild acute and chronic inflammation may be present within the superficial dermis and epithelium.

DIFFERENTIAL DIAGNOSIS

Erythematous vulvar candidiasis must be differentiated from Paget's disease, eczema, lichen simplex chronicus, psoriasis, and reactive vulvitis. Discovery of hyphae on KOH smears from the vagina and/or vulva will almost always resolve this point of differential diagnosis. Paget's disease is rarely as diffuse as vulvar candidiasis. Psoriasis will usually demonstrate a scaly appearance. Lichen simplex chronicus will be more hyperplastic and less diffuse. A reactive vulvitis will usually be associated with an antecedent history of recent use of, or exposure to, an irritative substance.

CLINICAL BEHAVIOR AND TREATMENT

Efforts to clear *Candida* vulvitis will be unsuccessful if the patient has undiagnosed and untreated diabetes mellitus. Persistence of vulvitis despite adequate therapy should prompt blood glucose evaluation and control of the blood glucose, if it is elevated. Patients who are taking recurrent or long-term antimicrobial therapy for extragenital disease should be forewarned that persistent and recurrent candidiasis may be a complication, and antifungal therapy should be instituted at the earliest notation of symptoms.

A useful agent for treating vulvar candidiasis is a combination of clotrimazole and betamethasone (Lotrisone cream). The steroid component of the topical cream will reduce inflammation and the desire to scratch while the clotrimazole exerts an antifungal activity. The cream should be used twice daily for approximately 2 weeks.

Numerous antifungal preparations exist to treat vaginal candidiasis and if these are ineffective, then consideration should be given to culturing for a re-sistent strain of fungus such as *Torulopsis glabrata*. Such infections may require topical application of gentian violet 1% solution or boric acid powder (600 mg in 0 gelatin capsules) intravaginally once daily for 10–14 days. With failure of topical therapies to alleviate recurrent candidiasis, consideration should be given to oral preparations such as fluconazole (Diflucan) and ketoconazole (Nizoral). Fluconazole may be started at 400 mg on the first day, followed by 200 mg daily on succeeding days. Ketoconazole may be administered as 200 mg daily. Therapy should be discontinued when cure is accomplished. Patients should be observed closely for evidence of hepatotoxicity, especially if therapy is prolonged.

Progressive Therapeutic Options

1. Treat vaginal candidiasis with over-the-counter antifungal vaginal preparations. Apply clotrimazole and betamethasone (Lotrisone) to the vulva twice daily for 10–14 days.
2. For recurrent disease (and a negative glucose screen, negative oral antibiotic history, and negative HIV screen):
   a) Gentian violet 1% painted on the vagina and vulva weekly for approximately three episodes. Patients should be forewarned that clothing may be stained and that occasionally a reactive vulvitis may be noted.
   b) Boric acid vaginal suppositories (600 mg in a 0 gelatin capsule) once or twice daily. Therapy may be continued for several weeks; however, irritative symptoms may prompt discontinuation.
   c) Oral fluconazole (Diflucan) at 400 mg once as initial dose, followed by 200 mg daily until symptoms resolve (2–4 weeks), or
   Oral ketoconazole (Nizoral) at 200 mg daily for 2–4 weeks.

NOTATION: If oral preparations are used for prolonged therapy, the possibility of hepatotoxicity increases and liver function test results should be followed closely.

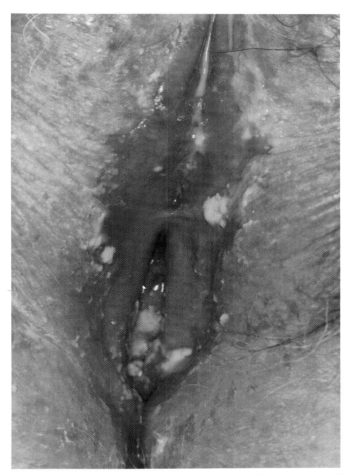

Figure 6.2. Diffuse erythematous changes observed in a patient with candida vulvovaginitis.

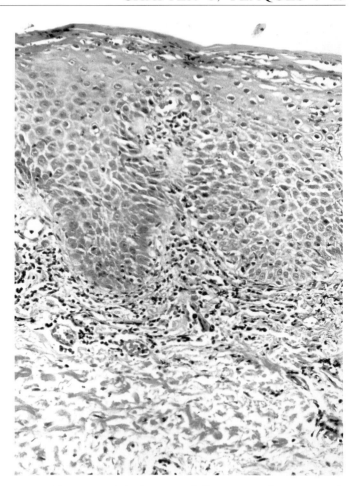

Figure 6.3. Fungal infection. Acute inflammatory cells are present in the superficial epithelium, where fungal organisms were identified.

Eczema (Atopic Dermatitis)

DEFINITION

Derived from the Greek word ekzein (to boil out), eczema is an inflammatory dermatologic disease, often of indeterminant etiology with acute, subacute, and chronic manifestations, most commonly presenting as a pruritic rash.

GENERAL FEATURES

Eczema may well be the most common inflammatory skin disease. The vulva is not a common site of eczema; however, pruritic vulvar rashes are common and an understanding of the evolution of acute eczema into chronic eczema is important for the clinician. Acute eczema is most commonly a manifestation of direct contact with an allergen. The classic example of this condition is the contact dermatitis noted after exposure to poison ivy. This process is self-limited; however, other allergens, either exogenous or endogenous, may result in a subacute inflammation, which eventually evolves into a chronic eczematous pattern associated with self-induced trauma secondary to intense scratching of pruritic vulvar skin. Often the inciting agent for the pruritus will remain unknown and indeed may be psychogenic.

CLINICAL PRESENTATION

The typical patient with vulvar eczema will present with complaints of intense vulvar pruritus. This discomfort may have been present for weeks to years. Rarely a patient exposed to an allergen such as poison ivy or poison oak will present in the acute phase complaining of pruritus, but the phase of acute eczema secondary to such contact is rarely seen. Most commonly the subacute and chronic phases of eczema will be observed by the clinician. Whereas acute eczema is a vesicular eruption associated with erythema, the subacute and chronic phases are associated with erythema and scale with nondescript borders. Persistence of inflammation and irritation, especially associated with scratching, will result in a plaquelike disease process with thickened skin and prominent skin markings. Rarely is it necessary to perform biopsy to arrive at a diagnosis.

MICROSCOPIC FINDINGS

The histopathologic features of atopic dermatitis, seborrhea dermatitis, dyshidrosis and atopic eczema are essentially identical. Acute spongiotic dermatitis with intraepidermal edema is an early feature and may be associated with vesicles. Subacute changes may be seen with a lymphocytic infiltrate within the epithelium, as well as in the papillary and superficial dermis. The diagnosis of contact (irritant) dermatitis should be considered if eosinophils are present. When the change is severe, allergic contact dermatitis should be considered.

ADJUNCTIVE STUDIES

No adjunctive studies are necessary to discern the etiology of this process.

DIFFERENTIAL DIAGNOSIS

The condition most commonly confused with eczema is psoriasis. Psoriasis generally has a much more intense erythema and discrete borders associated with silvery white scales. Psoriasis may also be found in rather characteristic extragenital areas such as the extensor surfaces of the elbows and knees and in prior incisional sites. Such findings would lend support to a diagnosis of psoriasis without the necessity to perform biopsy. Seborrhea may also be confused with eczema in the vulvar region. Seborrhea is particularly noted in such anatomic locations as the scalp, the face (eyebrows, nasolabial folds, ear canals and posterior auricular folds, and the presternal area). These areas will demonstrate a fine whitish scale over an erythematous base. Borders will appear nondescript. Often it may be impossible to differentiate on clinical grounds the rashes of eczema, psoriasis, and seborrhea.

CLINICAL BEHAVIOR AND TREATMENT

Acute eczema, secondary to contact allergy, requires control of pruritus primarily. This may be accomplished initially with cool, wet dressings containing Burow's solution. Antihistamines such as diphenhydramine (Benadryl) or hydroxyzine (Atarax) may be administered to relieve pruritus. Although topical steroid-containing creams may be applied to relieve itching, significantly greater relief may be obtained by administering oral prednisone in high doses for short periods of time. Twenty to 30 mg of prednisone taken twice daily for 7–10 days in adults will have significant antiinflammatory action and will contribute markedly to relief of the patient's pruritus. If evidence of infection is present (perhaps as a result of scratching), then oral antibiotics with activity against coagulase-producing staphylococci should be administered.

When dealing with a subacute or chronic eczema, efforts should be made to define an allergen and remove the allergen from contact with the patient's vulva. Such substances may be included in synthetic clothing materials, or perhaps feminine hygiene products. Patients may be advised to wear no undergarments until severe symptoms subside. Often this will result in significant relief of symptoms. Topical steroids such as medium-strength betamethasone 0.1% (Valisone) may be applied 2–3 times daily for 2 weeks with subsequent tapering of frequency of application. Weaker steroid preparations can then be used such as triamcinolone cream 0.1% (Kenalog). Ointments applied after showers or bathing will help seal in moisture and improve hydration of the skin. Lotions such as Keri lotion, Nutraderm, and NutraPlus may also be of assistance. Similar preparations are found in cream form. Soaps should be mild and hypoallergenic. Plaque-like chronic lesions unresponsive to topical steroids may require intralesional injection with triamcinolone acetonide (Kenalog 10).

Progressive Therapeutic Options

1. Hydration and lubrication of the skin with such creams and lotions as Keri, Nutraderm, or NutraPlus. Avoid frequent bathing with drying soaps and instead use hypoallergenic soaps such as Dove, Keri, or Lowilla.
2. For subacute and chronic eczema, topical steroids such as 0.1% betamethasone (Valisone) applied 2–3 times daily for 2 weeks with subsequent tapering to less frequent application or to a weaker steroid preparation such as triamcinolone 0.1% (Kenalog).
3. Antibiotic therapy directed against coagulase-producing staphylococcal organisms, if evidence of cellulitis is present (amoxicillin/clavulanate [Augmentin] 250 mg three times a day in non-penicillin-allergic patients.)
4. Intralesional injection of triamcinolone acetonide (Kenalog-10) with a small-gauge needle.

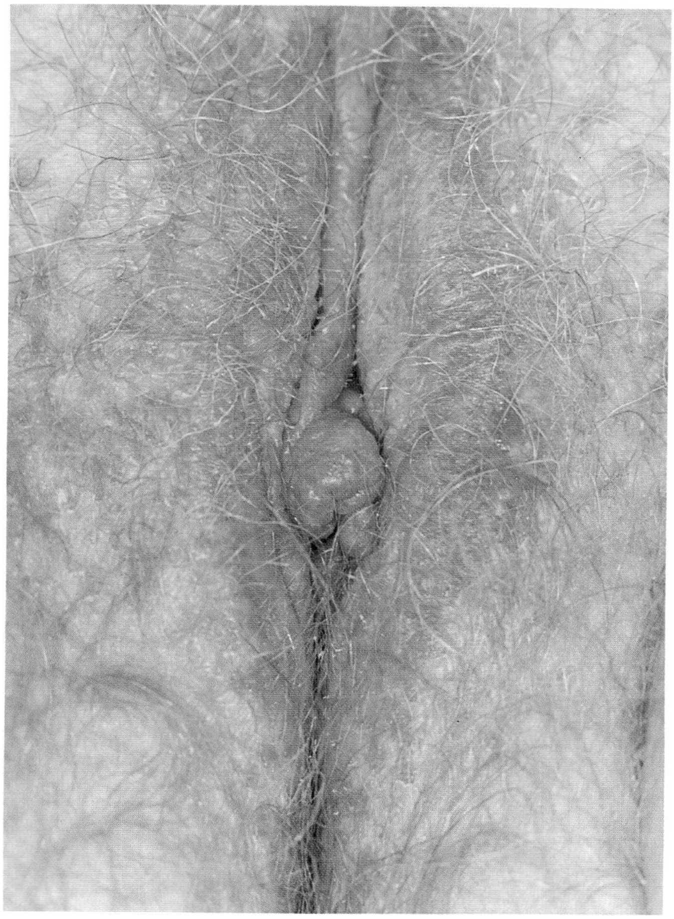

Figure 6.4. Moderate erythema in patient who complains of pruritus for 3 years. Clinical impression was eczema and patient was advised to use hypoallergenic soap. Condition resolved.

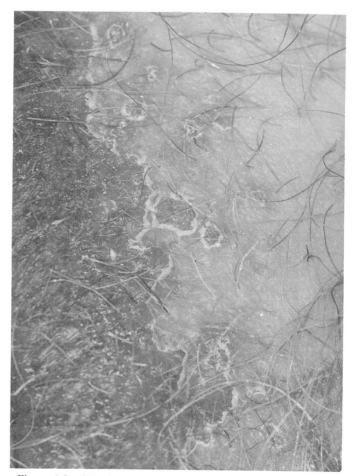

Figure 6.5. Note irregular border, erythema, and scaling of lesion.

Lichen Simplex Chronicus

DEFINITION

Lichen simplex chronicus is a chronic eczematous inflammation which results in thickened skin often associated with excoriation and fissures.

GENERAL FEATURES

Lichen simplex chronicus is observed most frequently in adults and may be related to stress. No known etiology for the condition has been determined, however, patients derive intense pleasure from scratching the extremely pruritic regions. This scratching leads to persistence of the localized area of inflammation.

CLINICAL PRESENTATION

Patients with vulvar lichen simplex chronicus will present complaining of moderate to severe pruritus, fairly well localized on the labial skin. This region will have been present for weeks or months. The patient will often describe an inability to sleep because of the intense desire to scratch the pruritic region. Scratching may lead to secondary infection.

MICROSCOPIC FINDINGS

Lichen simplex chronicus is charactered by thickening of the epithelium with acanthosis. Hyperkeratosis may be present. Within the superficial dermis, immediately beneath the epithelium, superficial dermal collagenization is present, which is typically associated with a deeper mild chronic inflammatory infiltrate. Superficial erosion with associated inflammatory cell exocytosis may be evident, secondary to scratching.

When inflammatory exocytosis is present, silver stain or periodic acid-Schiff is recommended to exclude fungal infection. If acanthosis is evident without dermal changes, the diagnosis of squamous cell hyperplasia is appropriate.

DIFFERENTIAL DIAGNOSIS

Conditions to be considered include psoriasis, candidiasis, and lichen sclerosus. Lesions seen with psoriasis are more sharply demarcated, and evidence of psoriasis may be present in extragenital locations such as the extensor surfaces of the arms. Candidal infections are of a more immediate duration than observed with lichen simplex chronicus. Usually there will be concomitant vaginal candidiasis. Lichen sclerosus patients will not demonstrate the scaly appearance that may be seen with lichen simplex chronicus, but an occasional lichen sclerosus patient will have adjacent squamous cell hyperplasia. Biopsy will be necessary to confirm the correct diagnosis and rule out atypia.

CLINICAL BEHAVIOR AND TREATMENT

Lichen simplex chronicus can be cured only if the itch-scratch cycle is terminated. Repetitive scratching leads to persistence of irritation and subsequent itching. Patients must be advised strongly to avoid scratching these lesions. Occasionally it may be necessary to have patients wear cotton gloves at bedtime to decrease trauma induced by subconscious scratching while asleep. If stress is a significant component of the patient's symptomatology, then emphasis should be placed upon alleviating this stress with behavioral modification. Extremely hypertrophied skin may require moderate to superpotent steroid application in the form of ointments. Moderate strength ointments such as betamethasone valerate 0.1% (Valisone) may be tried initially and if no response is noted a trial of a superpotent steroid such as clobetasol propionate 0.05% (Temovate) may be used for short periods of time. If no response is noted to topical applications of steroids, then it may be necessary to use intralesional injections of triamcinolone acetonide (Kenalog-10). If evidence of infection is present then oral antibiotics directed at common organisms such as staphylococci may be administered to decrease the infectious irritation.

Progressive Therapeutic Options

1. Topical steroid ointment with emphasis on lowest effective potency. For markedly hyperplastic skin it may be necessary to use moderate strength steroids such as betamethasone valerate 0.1% ointment (Valisone). Decrease to a lower strength steroid preparation after 2 weeks, especially if the condition involves the intertriginous folds.
2. Intense behavioral modification for patients demonstrating stress-related or stress-induced lichen simplex chronicus. In addition to counseling, patients must be advised not to scratch pruritic vulvar lesions.
3. Intralesional injection with triamcinolone acetonide (Kenalog-10).

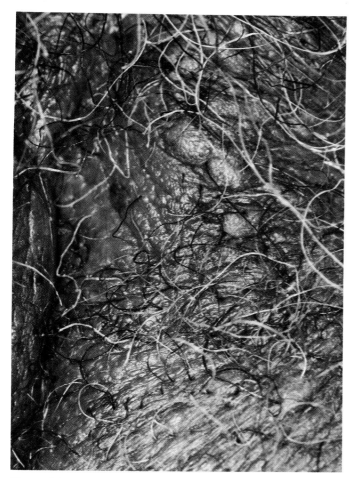

Figure 6.6. Hypertrophic vulvar skin in a 55-year-old woman with a 30-year history of pruritus. Biopsy confirmed clinical impression of lichen simplex chronicus; pruritus was relieved with Valisone 0.1% ointment.

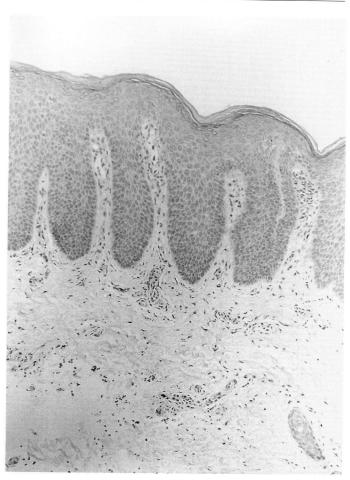

Figure 6.7. Lichen simplex chronicus. The acanthotic epithelium has markedly elongated and widened rete ridges. Spongiosis, with prominent intracellular bridges, is evident. There is collagenization of the underlying dermis with a superficial chronic inflammatory infiltrate immediately beneath the superficial collagized dermis.

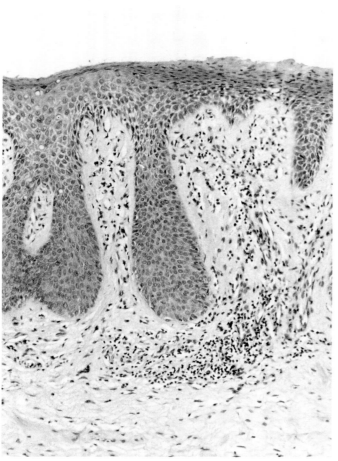

Figure 6.8. Lichen simplex chronicus. There is prominent acanthosis with deep and broad rete. A superficial inflammatory infiltrate is present in the dermis with a spared zone of dermis immediately beneath the basal layer.

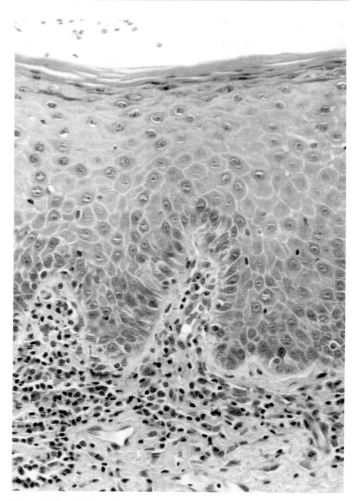

Figure 6.9. Lichen simplex chronicus. The epithelium is slightly thickened; however, no atypia is present. Within the superficial dermis, chronic inflammatory cells are present. The dermis immediately beneath the basal layer lacks inflammation and is fibrotic.

Paget's Disease

DEFINITION

Paget's disease is an intraepithelial neoplasia associated with proliferation of atypical glandular cells of apocrine type.

GENERAL FEATURES

Paget's disease is primarily a disease of postmenopausal women, most commonly caucasian women. The original description of Paget's disease pertained to breast adenocarcinoma. The later observation that Paget's disease could occur in extramammary locations, primarily the vulva, resulted in theories attributing the disease to glands in the "milk line." Although Paget's disease of the breast is always associated with adenocarcinoma of the breast, Paget's disease of the vulva is not usually associated with adenocarcinoma of the vulva. Fewer than 25% of cases will have underlying adenocarcinoma. Extravulvar carcinomas may be observed in patients with Paget's disease of the vulva. These carcinomas may be genital (vaginal, cervical, uterine), urologic (bladder), gastrointestinal (rectal or anorectal), or mammary (breast).

CLINICAL PRESENTATION

The usual patient with vulvar Paget's disease will be a woman presenting in her 60s with complaints of longstanding vulvar pruritus and discomfort. Although the disease has been reported in younger women and in the black population, this is exceedingly uncommon. On examination relatively discrete hyperplastic-appearing skin will be noted. There will be classically interspersed erythematous and excoriated areas alternating with patches of white epithelium. This process may be small (1–2 cm in diameter) or extensive, involving the entire labial and perianal skin.

MICROSCOPIC FINDINGS

Paget's disease is characterized by distinctive "Paget's cells" within the epithelium. These cells are typically as large as or larger than the adjacent keratinocytes. They are present singly and as clusters of cells throughout the epithelium with generally more cells, and larger groups of cells, present near the basal and parabasal layers. Paget cells have relatively large and prominent nucleoli. The cytoplasm is gray to blue gray on hematoxylin and eosin stain, and carcinoembryonic antigen and cytokeratin are immunoreactive. Paget's cells are often seen within the squamous epithelium of the adjacent skin appendages and hair shafts. This is a relatively common finding and should be discriminated from invasive Paget's disease.

Approximately 20% of patients with Paget's disease have associated adenocarcinoma. The adenocarcinoma may be arising from the overlying Paget disease; however, a more common finding is underlying adenocarcinoma arising from the Bartholin's gland or an adjacent sweat gland skin appendages. The underlying tumor will have the same immunoreactivity to carcinoembryonic antigen as the Paget's disease. When total examination of the vulvar epithelium involved with clinically evident Paget's disease demonstrates no underlying adenocarcinoma, deep local excision to the fascia is sufficient therapy. If adenocarcinoma is identified, bilateral inguinal-femoral lymphadenectomy is recommended.

As a general rule, it is not of value to perform frozen sections on the surgical margins in dealing with Paget's disease, nor is it clinically useful to perform carcinoembryonic antigen immunohistochemistry to detect occult Paget cells in the epithelium of the surgical margins. There is no recognized risk of associated underlying adenocarcinoma in normal-appearing areas peripheral to the clinically evident Paget's disease. Paget cells may be found remote from the clinically evident Paget's disease, in clinically normal-appearing epithelium. Radical total vulvectomy may not have free margins in such cases. A practical approach that conserves vulvar anatomy and reduces radical surgery, and the time and expense of frozen sections, is to follow the patient clinically; if clinical evidence of Paget's disease is found, treatment of those areas with local excision or laser vaporization is indicated, recognizing that such conservative therapy does not compromise the detection of adenocarcinoma, and that when the process is entirely intraepithelial, it is not life threatening.

ADJUNCTIVE STUDIES

Because of the association with extravulvar malignancy, the patient with vulvar Paget's disease should have an extensive evaluation before therapy. This should include vaginal and cervical cytology and colposcopy, endometrial biopsy, bladder cytology and cystoscopy, intravenous pyelography, barium studies and endoscopy of the gastrointestinal tract (especially of the lower gastrointestinal tract), and mammography.

DIFFERENTIAL DIAGNOSIS

The vulvar conditions most readily confused with Paget's disease include candidiasis, squamous cell intraepithelial neoplasia, eczema, and lichen sclerosus (especially the hyperplastic variety). Candidiasis is usually a much more diffuse process and the condition is typically associated with vaginal candidiasis. The diagnosis is confirmed with a KOH wet preparation. The patient will respond fairly rapidly to topical antifungal and steroid applications. Patients with vulvar intraepithelial neoplasia may also demonstrate well-circumscribed areas of hyperplastic-appearing skin. This skin will not typically demonstrate a weeping erythematous/white appearance. The diagnosis will require biopsy and pathologic review. Eczema may be seen in postmenopausal women and a variety of eczema, lichen simplex chronicus, may appear as a scaly, excoriated condition. The process may also be diffuse, involving both labia and the skin to the medial thighs. Histologic confirmation will be essential for final diagnosis. Hypertrophic lichen sclerosus will usually be observed in a field of parchmentlike lichen sclerosus. The patient may complain of pruritus, and excoriated skin due to scratching may pose a diagnostic dilemma for the clinician. Once again, biopsy will confirm the diagnosis.

CLINICAL BEHAVIOR AND TREATMENT

Untreated Paget's disease will continue to be symptomatic for the usual patient. Rarely will a patient be asymptomatic. Paget's disease has the potential for spreading vertically as well as horizontally and what begins as a localized process may spread, involving the entire vulva and perianal region. Given the association with an underlying adenocarcinoma, failure to diagnose and treat the process may result in metastatic disease and death. Likewise, failure to evaluate appropriately for extravulvar disease before initiating therapy may result in the progression of an undiagnosed breast, bladder, cervical, or bowel carcinoma.

The major step in evaluating patients with Paget's disease does not involve the use of a colposcope or toluidine blue. It involves careful palpation of the vulvar lesion. Underlying masses, nodularity, or fibrosis may well be indicative of an associated underlying adenocarcinoma and this observation warrants deep biopsy of this tissue. If histology of an underlying nodule or fibrosis indicates adenocarcinoma, the patient should be counseled for a radical vulvectomy to determine presence of nodal spread. With nodal metastasis the prognosis is poor. The place of adjuvant chemotherapy and radiotherapy has not been adequately defined and results are primarily anecdotal. If the patient has no underlying apocrine adenocarcinoma, then therapy is surgical and involves wide, local excision of the disease process. The margin of the obvious disease process should be demarcated in the operating room. Two to three centimeters of clinically disease-free skin (and the lesion) should be excised in a circumferential fashion and clearly oriented before submission to pathology. It should be remembered that Paget's disease may migrate vertically as well as horizontally and the excised specimen should involve the entire skin thickness into the subcuticular adipose tissue to assure removal of all skin appendages. The defect may be closed primarily, covered with a skin graft, or allowed to heal secondarily.

Despite all efforts to excise Paget's disease of the vulva, disease may recur and patients should be followed carefully. Any area of pruritus or obvious excoriation should be removed. Although laser therapy and other destructive approaches have been used, local excision will provide valuable information regarding diagnosis and the presence or absence of associated adenocarcinoma.

Progressive Therapeutic Options

1. With no evidence of an underlying apocrine gland carcinoma, wide local excision should be accomplished with 2–3 cm clear margins of resection, with excision to the fascia.
2. With evidence of an underlying apocrine gland carcinoma, a radical vulvectomy with associated regional inguinal femoral node resection should be accomplished. Adjuvant chemotherapy and radiotherapy issues should be discussed with the appropriate specialist. Results are primarily anecdotal.
3. Careful follow-up examinations and excision of any areas suggestive of recurrent disease.

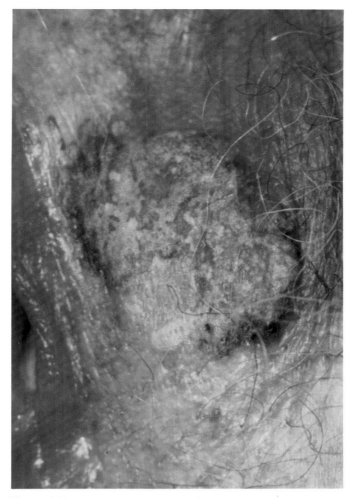

Figure 6.10. Paget's disease of the left labium majus treated by wide local excision. One margin was involved in the periclitoral region (illustration compliments of Dr. Mark Gelder).

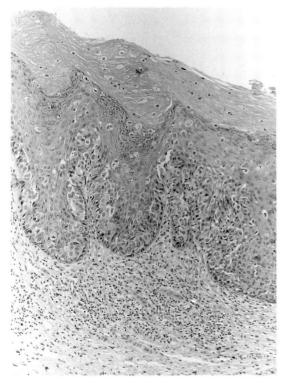

Figure 6.11. Paget's disease. Paget cells are present in the basal and parabasal areas. A few isolated Paget cells are in the superficial epithelium.

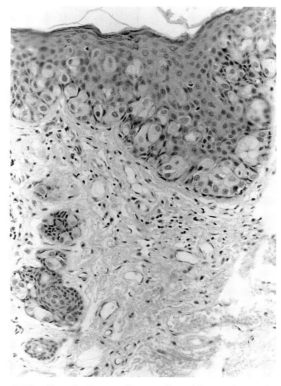

Figure 6.12. Paget's disease. Paget cells, with prominent clear cytoplasm, are evident throughout the epithelium.

Plasma Cell Vulvitis (Vulvitis Circumscripta Plasma Cellularis)

DEFINITION

Plasma cell vulvitis is a chronic, inflammatory process involving the vestibule and labia minora that results in an erythematous, almost velvety-appearing lesion.

GENERAL FEATURES

Plasma cell vulvitis is a rare entity that may be considered analogous to plasma cell balanitis of Zoon, which was originally described on the penile shaft. Cytologic criteria for the diagnosis have varied between observers but have generally included epidermal thinning, with a marked plasma cell infiltrate. Some have believed plasma cell vulvitis to be a variant of lichen planus.

CLINICAL PRESENTATION

The patient will present with pain or pruritus at the vulvar introitus. On examination, a velvety, reddish lesion will be apparent. The condition may be extensive, involving a major portion of the vestibule, or may be somewhat localized to smaller areas in this region.

MICROSCOPIC FINDINGS

Plasma cell vulvitis is characterized by a lichenoid inflammatory infiltrate that consists primarily of plasma cells. The involved epithelium is typically thinned with thinning of the rete ridges. Prominent epithelial spongiosis is associated with horizontally oriented parabasal cells, which are considered helpful in establishing the microscopic diagnosis. The epithelial surface is not keratinized nor is a granular layer evident. The submucosal or dermal inflammatory infiltrate extends perivascularly about dilated dermal vessels. Interdermal extravascular blood and hemosiderin may be seen about these vessels. Microscopically the perivascular inflammatory infiltrate must be distinguished from syphilis. Other chronic dermatoses, especially lichen planus, must be considered.

DIFFERENTIAL DIAGNOSIS

With extensive disease the differential diagnosis would include such conditions as psoriasis, eczema, or lichen planus. Psoriasis and eczema would rarely involve the vestibule and are more commonly seen in the pilosebaceous region of the vulva. Lichen planus is rarely limited to the vestibule. It more commonly presents as a desquamative inflammatory vaginitis. Additionally, one must consider such possibilities as cicatricial pemphigoid, pemphigus, and autoimmune diseases that affect mucosal surfaces. Immunohistology will be of assistance in differentiating these. Although vulvar intraepithelial neoplasia is usually not erythematous, it, too, should be considered in the differential. The observation of velvety red appearing tissue in the region of the vestibule should immediately suggest the possibility of plasma cell vulvitis. A biopsy should be obtained for a confirmation of the diagnosis.

CLINICAL BEHAVIOR AND TREATMENT

Symptoms may be controlled with topical steroids if pruritus is a major component. Topical steroids such as betamethasone 0.1% applied as an ointment may result in significant alleviation of the patient's discomfort; however, the disease is extremely recalcitrant to therapeutic intervention.

Progressive Therapeutic Option

1. Topical steroid applications (betamethasone 0.1% ointment).
2. Superficial laser ablation of the involved epithelium has been employed; however, there is little experience with this approach.

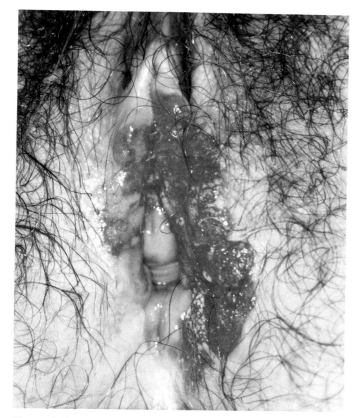

Figure 6.13. Plasma cell vulvitis. A red, erosive-appearing lesion occupies the vulvar vestibule, medial aspects of the labia minora, and a portion of the perineal body (photo courtesy of Dr. Frits B. Lammes, Amsterdam, The Netherlands).

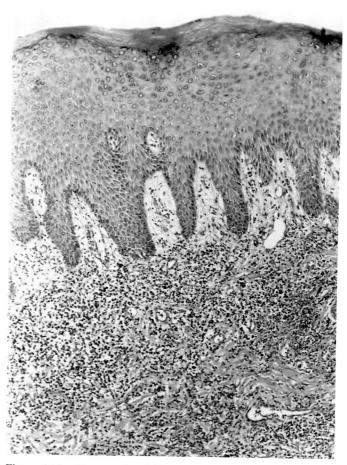

Figure 6.14. Plasma cell vulvitis. There is a dense chronic inflammatory infiltrate within the superficial and deeper dermis consisting predominately of plasma cells. The epithelium is thickened and spongiotic.

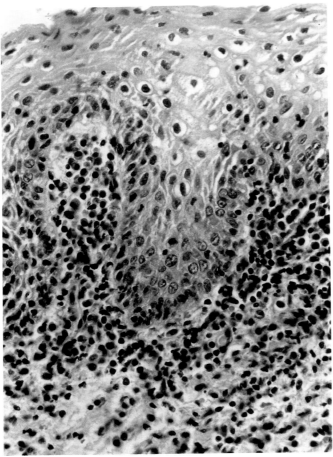

Figure 6.15. Plasma cell vulvitis. The epithelial spongiosis is associated with fusiform (lozenge-shaped) keratinocytes. The plasma cell rich infiltrate involves the epithelial dermal interface.

Psoriasis

DEFINITION

Psoriasis is a papulosquamous dermatosis characterized by erythematous papules and plaques typically covered with white or silvery scales.

GENERAL FEATURES

This condition is seen in 1–2% of the population and is presumed to be multifactorial in inheritance. The etiology is not defined.

CLINICAL PRESENTATION

The typical patient with psoriasis exhibits pink to red plaques with white scale on the extensor surfaces of the elbows and knees, the lumbar region, and the scalp. Identical lesions are observed on the vulva and may be so confluent and widespread as to mimic candidiasis, tinea cruris, or cellulitis. Pruritus may be present, and is often the presenting complaint. Psoriasis may be associated with onycholysis and pitting of the nails, annulus migrans of the tongue (annular, raised lesions), inflammatory bowel disease, and arthritis. Disease activity may directly relate to stress levels.

The diagnosis of psoriasis rarely requires a biopsy. The typical lesions will be seen in the usual distribution. Occasionally, the vulvar condition may appear to be inflamed and extensive, and lesions elsewhere may appear to be quiescent. Clinical signs that may be of help include (a) Koebner reaction, occurrence of new lesions of psoriasis at sites of skin injury; (b) Woronoff's ring, blanching skin immediately surrounding a psoriatic plaque; and (c) Auspitz's sign, bleeding sites occurring after removal of a psoriatic scale. If candidiasis is a distinct possibility, then a KOH preparation of desquamated scrapings may be examined for typical hyphae. In patients in whom the diagnosis is uncertain, biopsy is indicated.

MICROSCOPIC FINDINGS

The histopathologic findings of psoriasis include uniform acanthosis, with elongation of the rete ridges to a similar length. Small aggregates of acute inflammatory cells are present within the epithelium, forming intraepithelial abscesses (Munro abscesses). Hyperkeratosis and parakeratosis are typically evident; however, there is usually a decreased granular layer. Epithelial mitotic activity is typically increased. Within the superficial dermis, there is a mild chronic inflammatory infiltrate. The dermal papillae are elongated, and broadened or "clubbed" between the elongated rete ridges.

ADJUNCTIVE STUDIES

No additional studies are necessary.

DIFFERENTIAL DIAGNOSIS

The differential diagnosis of an erythematous vulva includes candidiasis, eczema, Paget's disease, seborrhea, and possibly secondary syphilis. All of these conditions may create plaquelike lesions. Psoriasis is rather unique in its presentation as a deep-red, sharply demarcated vulvar lesion. Seborrhea and eczema may appear as red lesions; however, their borders are less well defined. The classic location of psoriasis on extensor surfaces and in prior incision sites would help to differentiate it from seborrhea. Seborrhea is more classically seen in areas of sebum production, such as the edge of the scalp, the nasolabial folds and the presternal area. Candidiasis will present as a wide-spread vulvar erythema that may be as intense as that seen with psoriasis. Candidiasis will not have scales but rather may have an attached fungal exudate. KOH preparation will help differentiate this condition. The raised, sometimes reddish, lesions of secondary syphilis are moist and exuberant. Paget's disease is not associated with scaling. Lichen planus may present as an erythematous process but usually the erythema is confined to the vestibule and vagina without extension onto the vulva. There will not be scaling noted with lichen planus.

CLINICAL BEHAVIOR AND TREATMENT

Therapy is tailored to the extent and severity of the disease. Minor vulvar psoriasis in the pilosebaceous area may be treated with a local tar application. Tar shampoos (Denorex, Tegrin, Neutrogena) used regularly in the pubic hair often will control the scaling.

Short contact application with anthralin cream may be efficacious for chronic plaques; however, patients must be forewarned that temporary staining of the skin and permanent staining of clothing may be problematic. Initiate therapy with anthralin (Dithrocreme) 0.1% and apply once daily for 1 week. Remove after approximately 20–30 minutes and bathe to decrease staining and irritation. Gradual increases at weekly intervals in strength of anthralin may be accomplished (0.25%, 0.5%, 1.0%) based on response and lack of irritation. Avoid the intertriginous areas to decrease inflammatory reaction.

The most commonly used topical preparations for vulvar psoriasis contain steroids. Selection of the appropriate steroid should be based on the extent of the psoriasis. It may be appropriate to use superpotent steroids such as halobetasol 0.05% (Ultravate) or clobetasol 0.05% (Temovate) for a hyperkeratotic localized lesion of psoriasis. With improvement in the lesion, superpotent steroids should be discontinued after 2 weeks of twice-daily use. Therapy may be reinstated if needed after 1–2 weeks of recovery. Application of superpotent steroids to large areas of vulvar psoriasis may result in significant absorption of the steroid and adrenal suppression. For more extensive areas of psoriasis, medium- or low-potency steroids are more appropriate. Avoid use of superpotent steroids in skin creases. Less potent compounds tend to create less atrophy (hydrocortisone 0.1%, triamcinolone 0.1%). Small plaques may respond remarkably to a single intralesional injection of triamcinolone (Kenalog-5 or -10).

Vitamin D analogs (0.005% calcipotriene [Dovonex]) may be as efficacious as betamethasone 0.1% and short-contact anthralin in managing psoriasis. Application is accomplished twice daily, avoiding flexures and not exceeding 100 g/week. The possibility for alteration in calcium metabolism exists and if it is necessary to use more than 100 g of analog weekly, serum calcium levels should be monitored.

Phototherapy has been used extensively for psoriasis. It is more readily used in regions other than the vulva. The mechanism of action is poorly understood but relates to vitamin D metabolism. Phototherapy may be combined with the use of 1–5% cold tar (Goeckerman therapy). It may also be combined with the use of anthralin (Ingram method). Alternatively, phototherapy may be augmented with oral or topical psoralens (PUVA therapy). Concern exists that long-term phototherapy may induce squamous cell carcinoma.

Extensive psoriasis unresponsive to topical agents may require the use of systemic therapy. The decision to use systemic therapy should be based upon the severity of the disease. Options include methotrexate, retinoids (etretinate), and cyclosporine. All of these regimens have the potential for significant side effects and their use is warranted only for treatment of the most severe forms of psoriasis.

Throughout the period of pharmacologic intervention to control vulvar psoriasis, emphasis must be placed on controlling stress levels.

Progressive Therapeutic Options

1. Behavioral modification to decrease stress.
2. For minor vulvar disease;
   a) Tar shampoos (Denorex, Tegrin, Neutrogena) to the pubic hair.
   b) Low (hydrocortisone 0.1%) to moderate (betamethasone 0.1%) strength steroid ointments or creams for short-term use.
   c) Intralesional triamcinolone (Kenalog 5 or 10) for small, discrete plaques in minimal numbers and of a chronic nature.
3. For moderate vulvar disease:
   a) Trial of anthralin cream (Dithrocreme) 0.1% twice a day for 1 week (remove after 20–30 minutes followed by bathing). Increase strength (0.25%, 0.5%, 1.0%) at weekly intervals, as tolerated. Avoid intertriginous areas and warn about staining.
   b) Superpotent steroids (halobetasol, clobetasol) twice daily for 2 weeks followed by a rest cycle of 1–2 weeks.
   c) Vitamin D analog (0.005% calcipotriene) twice daily, not to exceed 100 g weekly
4. For severe vulvar disease unresponsive to previous regimens:
   a) Consider retinoids (etretinate) for pustular and erythrodermic psoriasis. Plaquelike psoriasis is less responsive. Careful counseling concerning teratogenicity and absolute need for contraception. Careful monitoring of liver function tests, complete blood cell count, cholesterol, triglycerides.
   b) Consider methotrexate.
   c) Consider cyclosporine.

NOTATION: Use of methotrexate or cyclosporine requires familiarity with short-term and long-term toxicity. Severity of disease must warrant potential risks.

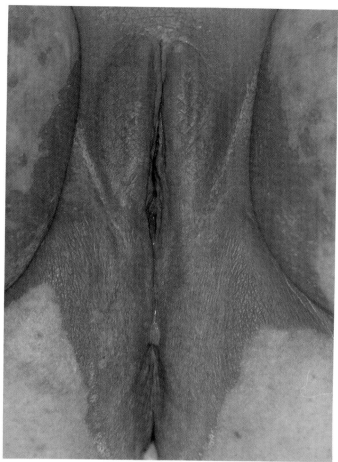

Figure 6.16. Psoriasis in a pregnant patient at 30 weeks' gestation. Noted marked erythema, sharply demarcated borders, and satellite lesions.

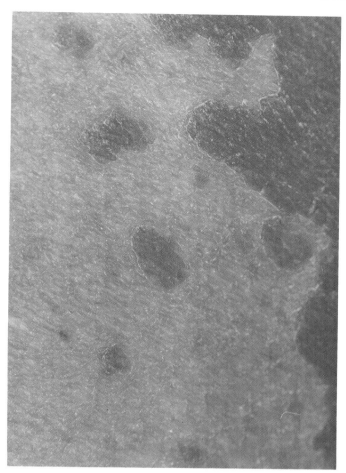

Figure 6.17. Magnified view of sharply demarcated borders and marked erythema.

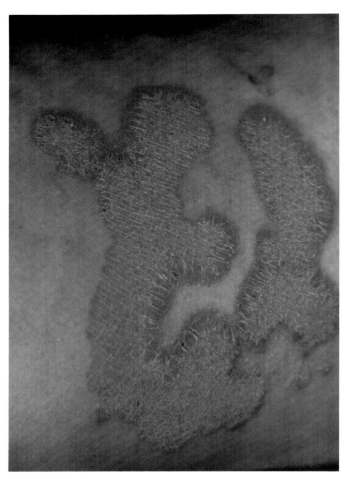

Figure 6.18. Silvery white scale observed on psoriatic plaques.

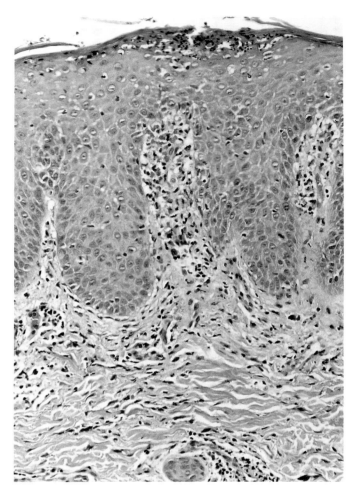

Figure 6.19. Psoriasis. The keratin layer is partially disrupted and the epithelium is acanthotic with elongated and widened rete ridges. A superficial intraepithelial abscess containing acute inflammatory cells is present.

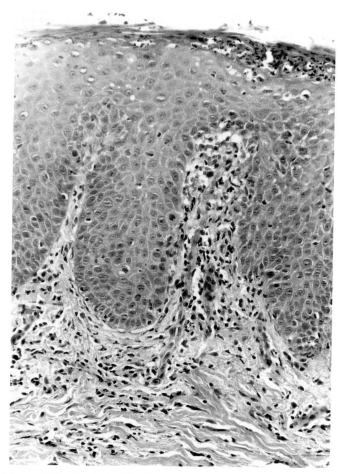

Figure 6.20. Psoriasis. The Munro microabscess is present within the superficial epithelium.

Seborrhea

DEFINITION

Seborrhea is a chronic inflammatory disease associated with a characteristic distribution in areas of sebum production, particularly the face and scalp.

GENERAL FEATURES

Seborrhea may be observed in all age groups, affecting infants (cradle cap), young children (blepharitis), and adults (classic seborrhea). Vulvar involvement with seborrhea is uncommon, yet may be observed in patients with or without classic extragenital seborrhea. The etiology is unknown and may be a consequence of increased sebum production secondary to increased sensitivity to androgens. Alternatively, local infection with fungal organisms may incite this chronic dermatitis. Stress and emotional strain may be important etiologic agents in the development of seborrhea.

CLINICAL PRESENTATION

Patients usually will present complaining of pruritus of the vulva. Scratching may result in significant irritation and secondary cellulitis. On examination a diffuse erythematous rash will be noted. The lesion is usually symmetric. Careful examination may demonstrate a fine scale over the erythematous base. Extragenital involvement will usually be noted in the scalp (particularly at the margins of the scalp), the nasolabial folds, the external ear canal, the posterior auricular fold, the eyebrows, the base of the eyelashes, and the sternal region. Presence of a similar rash in these regions is classic for seborrhea and the clinician may take relative assurance that this is the appropriate diagnosis. It is rare that biopsy will be necessary to define the diagnosis of seborrhea.

MICROSCOPIC FEATURES

Seborrhea (seborrheic dermatitis) is a spongiotic dermatitis characterized by spongiosis, which is typically not severe, acanthosis, and focal parakeratosis. In untreated cases the parakeratosis may be focal, immediately adjacent to the hair follicles. A mild chronic inflammatory cell infiltrate is usually present within the dermis, associated with focal inflammatory cell exocytosis. In patients with a long-standing history of self-treatment, overriding contact dermatitis changes may be present and eosinophils may be within the inflammatory cell infiltrate.

ADJUNCTIVE STUDIES

No adjunctive studies are necessary to evaluate seborrhea. Diffuse disease may be seen in immunocompromised patients and such a finding may warrant HIV screening.

DIFFERENTIAL DIAGNOSIS

The primary lesions involved in the differential diagnosis of seborrhea are eczema and psoriasis. Psoriasis has a much more discrete border and a white, silvery scale. Psoriasis is seen on the extensor surfaces of the arms and legs and in the prior incision sites. Seborrhea is not seen in these locations. Differentiation from eczema is often difficult and may be a moot point because both conditions may be treated similarly.

CLINICAL BEHAVIOR AND TREATMENT

Seborrhea is a chronic recurring condition. It may be exacerbated during periods of stress. Efforts should be made to minimize stress with behavioral modification. Pilosebaceous areas of the vulva may be shampooed with selenium sulfide (Selsen or Selsen Blue). Sulfur and salicylic acid shampoos such as Sebulex may be used. Topical low- to medium-strength steroids may be applied such as triamcinolone acetonide 0.1% (Kenalog) or betamethasone valerate 0.1% (Valisone). Persistent and resistent cases of seborrhea may be managed with ketoconazole cream (Nizoral cream) applied twice daily for approximately 4 weeks.

Progressive Therapeutic Options

1. Behavioral modification to reduce stress.
2. Daily shampooing with selenium sulfide solutions (Selsen or Selsen Blue) or sulfur and salicylic acid shampoos (Sebulex).
3. Topical application of low- to medium-strength corticosteroid creams such as 0.1% triamcinolone acetonide (Kenalog), fluocinolone acetonide 0.25% (Synalar), or betamethasone valerate 0.1% (Valisone).
4. Ketoconazole 2% cream (Nizoral) applied twice daily for 4 weeks.

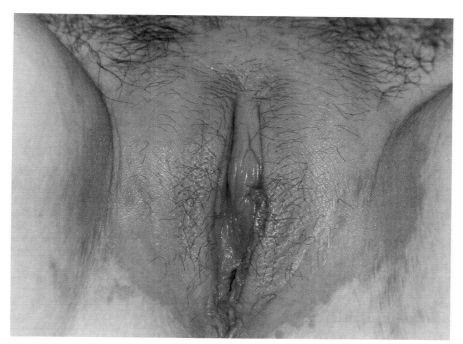

Figure 6.21. Classic "oily"-appearing skin of seborrhea noted in a patient with similar lesions in the scalp and nasolabial folds. Vulvar condition was exacerbated after the patient received implantable contraception (Levonorgestrel). Note the loss of pubic hair related to excess sebum production.

Squamous Cell Hyperplasia

DEFINITION

Squamous cell hyperplasia is a nonspecific thickening of vulvar epithelium characterized by acanthosis without a prominent inflammatory component. Hyperkeratosis may be present.

GENERAL FEATURES

This condition is rarely seen on the vulva. It may be a consequence of exposure to an irritating or inflammatory agent such as laundry products or occlusive underwear fabrics. Usually the inciting agent will remain undetermined.

CLINICAL PRESENTATION

Pruritus is the usual presenting symptom. On examination plaquelike, white epithelium will be noted. The contour will be irregular. The disease is usually unilateral. Confirmation of diagnosis will require biopsy.

MICROSCOPIC FINDINGS

The histopathologic diagnosis of squamous cell hyperplasia is a diagnosis of exclusion. Pathologic changes include prominent acanthosis with elongation, widening and deepening of the rete ridges and thickening of the epidermis. Hyperkeratosis may be present but there is no epithelial atypia. A mild, chronic, inflammatory infiltrate may be noted in the dermis. The term squamous cell hyperplasia encompasses changes previously specified as hyperplastic dystrophy but should not be used in the presence of a specific dermatosis (i.e., psoriasis, lichen planus, lichen simplex chronicus). Certain monilial and dermatophyte infections may demonstrate similar epithelial changes and should be excluded. Those cases demonstrating atypia should be classified as vulvar intraepithelial neoplasia.

ADJUNCTIVE STUDIES

No studies are indicated.

DIFFERENTIAL DIAGNOSIS

Plaquelike white epithelium on the vulva may be consistent with a hyperplastic variety of lichen sclerosus. In such cases there will be the usual stigmata of lichen sclerosus observed diffusely around the hyperplastic epithelium. There will be agglutination of the labia minora and often complete obliteration of the clitoris. Histologic specimens will demonstrate changes consistent with lichen sclerosus.

Plaquelike white epithelium may also be noted in patients with vulvar intraepithelial neoplasia. This process will usually be multifocal, although not invariably. Examination of the vulva after 5% acetic acid application and visualization through colposcope will demonstrate this multifocal pattern. Biopsy will confirm the diagnosis.

CLINICAL BEHAVIOR AND TREATMENT

Treatment of squamous cell hyperplasia is directed at control of pruritus. Topical steroids will be the mainstay of therapy. Betamethasone (Valisone) 0.1% ointment will almost invariably control symptoms. The ointment may be applied twice daily until symptoms are controlled, usually in 10–14 days. Use thereafter will be episodic. If the medium-strength steroids fail to control symptoms, then high-potency topical steroids such as clobetasol (Temovate) may be applied. Rarely will it be necessary to inject triamcinolone acetonide (Kenalog-10). Efforts should be made to determine what agents may be the etiologic factors in development of the squamous cell hyperplasia. Alterations in laundry products and avoidance of synthetic underwear may be of assistance.

Progressive Therapeutic Options

1. Apply medium-strength steroid ointments such as betamethasone 0.1% ointment (Valisone) twice daily until pruritus is controlled.
2. High-potency topical steroids such as clobetasol (Temovate) applied twice daily until symptoms are controlled and then tapered to sparing use of a less potent steroid.

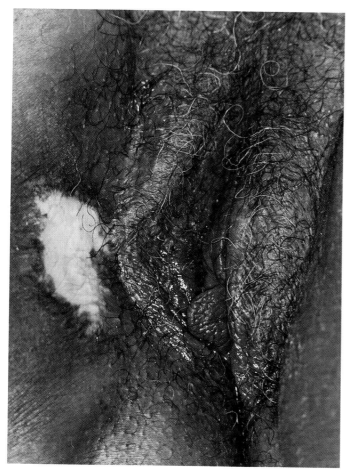

Figure 6.22. Pruritic, hypertrophied plaque of squamous cell hyperplasia, managed with Valisone 0.1% ointment with resolution of symptoms.

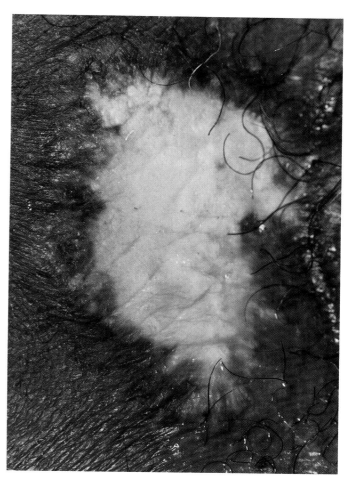

Figure 6.23. Magnified view of plaque of squamous cell hyperplasia, biopsy confirmed.

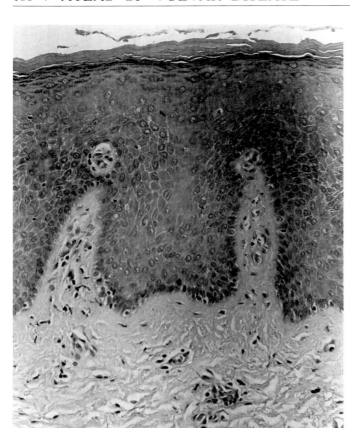

Figure 6.24. Squamous cell hyperplasia. The epithelium is thickened and acanthotic with a keratinized surface. No significant collagenization or inflammation is present within dermis.

Vulvar Intraepithelial Neoplasia (VIN)

DEFINITION

VIN is a proliferative intraepithelial squamous process characterized by abnormal epithelial maturation, nuclear enlargement, and nuclear atypia. Based upon the extent of replacement of epithelium by abnormal cells, VIN is categorized as VIN 1 (mild dysplasia), VIN 2 (moderate dysplasia), or VIN 3 (severe dysplasia/carcinoma in situ). The term vulvar intraepithelial neoplasia replaces such previously used terms as Bowen's disease, erythroplasia of Queyrat, carcinoma simplex, and Bowenoid papulosis.

GENERAL FEATURES

There appears to be an increasing incidence of vulvar intraepithelial neoplasia, especially in younger women. There is a strong association between disease occurrence and human papillomavirus, especially type 16, which has been identified in approximately 80% of VIN 3 specimens.

CLINICAL PRESENTATION

Most commonly patients with symptomatic vulvar intraepithelial neoplasia will complain of vulvar pruritus and superficial dyspareunia. Vulvar inspection reveals maculopapular lesions with color changes ranging from white to red to dark shades of brown. The lighter lesions may suggest a diagnosis of condylomata acuminata and the darker lesions may seem consistent with junctional or compound nevi. Occasionally no lesions will be noted upon vulvar examination and it will be necessary to evaluate the vulva with the colposcope after application of 5% acetic acid. Small, white lesions may then be noted in the vulvar and/or perianal skin. These lesions will usually be multicentric. Thorough examination of the vulva, vestibule, and perianal skin is always mandatory in all VIN patients. As many as 50% of patients with VIN may have anal involvement. Thorough examination of the vagina and cervix is also warranted because of the multicentricity of intraepithelial neoplasia in the lower reproductive tract.

The diagnosis of vulvar intraepithelial neoplasia is suspected based upon visual inspection and magnified colposcopic inspection of the vulva. Although toluidine blue has been used to accentuate neoplastic epithelium, the test is flawed by uptake of toluidine in inflammatory epithelium, which has been denuded or irritated by scratching. A more appropriate evaluation of the vulva is accomplished via colposcopy. The entire vulva should be observed after application of 5% acetic acid. The patient may apply this to the vulva on a cloth for several minutes before the colposcopic examination. Representative biopsies should be obtained from multicentric areas of abnormality. Special concern should be exercised to biopsy markedly hyperplastic or ulcerative lesions. Extensive biopsies should be obtained to exclude the possibility of invasive carcinoma within large fields of intraepithelial neoplasia. The progression of VIN to invasive carcinoma occurs in probably fewer than 15% of cases; however, the natural history is poorly defined because of the tendency to treat the disease rather than follow it. As has been noted with early stages of cervical intraepithelial neoplasia, early VIN may regress without therapy. Approximately 10% of patients with VIN 3 have been noted to have contiguous vulvar squamous cell carcinoma.

MICROSCOPIC FINDINGS

VIN is characterized by disorderly keratinocyte maturation associated with nuclear hyperchromasia, varying degrees of pleomorphism, and disordered and vertical orientation of the involved keratinocytes. Keratinocyte crowding and disorder within the basal layer are seen in all cases. Mitotic activity may be evident in the mid- and superficial epithelium, and the mitosis may be of abnormal configuration or dispersed. Depending upon the extent of disorderly maturation, the VIN may be graded 1 to 3, with VIN 1 representing disordered maturation in the lower one-third of the epithelium, VIN 2 representing disorderly growth in the lower two-thirds of the epithelium, and VIN 3 being interpreted in cases with more than the lower two-thirds of the epithelium having disordered growth. These findings are summarized in Table 6.1.

VIN lesions may have variable degrees of dyskeratosis. Hyperkeratosis and/or parakeratosis may be evident. Small "dyskeratotic" cells with prominent eosinophilic cytoplasm may be evident, representing aggregated tonofilaments with individual keratinocytes.

Three morphologic types of VIN are now recognized, namely basaloid, warty, and well-differentiated types. Basaloid VIN is characterized by relatively small, crowded basal-type keratinocytes that lack maturation and have coarse hyperchromatic nuclear chromatin. Warty VIN has koilocytosis, multinucleated keratinocytes, and other features of condyloma acuminatum, but lacks the cellular uniformity and evident maturation, as seen in the typical condyloma acuminatum. Warty VIN may have prominent hyperkeratosis and parakeratosis as well as "dyskeratotoic" keratinocytes. Basaloid and warty VIN may be found concurrently in a given patient, or may, on occasion, be evident in the same lesion, with transition from one cell type to another. Both types are recognized to be associated with human papillomavirus (HPV), especially HPV type 16.

Well-differentiated VIN is relatively uncommon and is characterized by increased eosinophilic cytoplasm and dyskeratosis within the basal and parabasal keratinocytes, usually evident at the deep tip of the rete ridges. The involved keratinocytes have relatively large nuclei compared with the more superficial cells, with vesicular chromatin and prominent nucleoli. This pattern of cellular change is commonly seen associated with vulvar squamous cell carcinoma. Well-differentiated VIN should be classified as VIN 3 and a search for associated invasive carcinoma should be made.

In non-hair-bearing skin, VIN averages approximately 1 mm in thickness; however, in hair-bearing skin, VIN may involve hair follicles and the ducts of sebaceous glands and in this situation may exceed 2.3 mm from the surface. Skin appendage involvement should be discriminated from superficial invasion. When this differential arises, deeper sections into the block bearing the area in question will usually resolve the issue. With skin appendage involvement, deeper contiguous sebaceous gland or hair-shaft epithelium will be evident. The cells along the basal layer maintain their palisaded orientation and do not protrude into the stroma. A localized stromal inflammatory cell infiltrate, or desmoplastic stromal response, is absent, as is usually seen with invasive tumor.

Approximately 15% of VIN lesions are pigmented. On biopsy, melanin can be found in the basal keratinocytes and within some of the superficial dermal macrophages. Dendritic melanocytes may be evident in the basal layer. VIN lesions from normally pigmented skin are often pigmented, whereas those from the vulvar vestibule are rarely pigmented. VIN lesions involving the vestibule are often red to pink and often resemble squamous intraepithelial lesions arising near the ectocervix or vagina.

CLINICAL BEHAVIOR AND TREATMENT

Treatment of vulvar intraepithelial neoplasia will be based upon the extent and severity of the disease. For isolated lesions of VIN appropriately evaluated by extensive colposcopy, excisional biopsy may be performed in the clinic, and this will be both diagnostic and therapeutic. An appropriate margin should be obtained. Cases with positive margins may have a recurrence rate of 20% or greater. Multicentric disease is difficult to manage in an office setting and will require either laser therapy or excision in the operating room. One must be certain that invasive disease has been excluded by extensive histologic sampling before performing laser ablation of vulvar intraepithelial neoplasia. Laser ablation is accomplished under appropriate anesthesia with power densities of 500–1000 watts/cm². To decrease lateral thermal damage, intermittent cooling of the vulva with ice packs may be helpful. Laser ablation should be accomplished in pilosebaceous skin to the third surgical plane, which is defined histologically as the midreticular dermis. It is necessary to obtain this plane of destruction to destroy neoplasia that may be present in the sebaceous glands and pilosebaceous ducts associated with hair follicles. Persistence of disease within these ducts will lead to a high rate of recurrence. This plane of laser ablation is recognized after destruction of the superficial epidermis and papillary dermis and is apparent when one visualizes collagen bundles, appearing as grayish to white fibers, present within the reticular dermis. In the pilosebaceous region of the vulva this zone is approximately 2.5 mm from the surface epithelium. If extensive histologic sampling before laser ablation has demonstrated deep involvement of the pilosebaceous ducts, a more appropriate approach would be excision of the involved area and submission to pathology. The laser may be used to augment surgical excision by destroying areas of vulvar intraepithelial neoplasia in the nonpilosebaceous areas, such as the vestibule and labia minora. These areas, highlighted by applying 5% acetic acid before laser ablation, should be destroyed, preferably by using colposcopically directed laser ablation. After completion of the laser ablation, Silvadene cream may be applied to the vulva and the patient may be discharged with oral analgesic therapy. She should be advised to use sitz baths daily and salt solutions may be added to the water to ameliorate her discomfort. If the laser ablation is taken to the base of the third surgical plane and has entered the adipose tissue, the resultant full-thickness burn will take weeks to heal. If the destruction is widespread, skin grafts may be required to effect skin continuity. Deep laser ablation should be avoided.

Patients with multicentric disease and deep pilosebaceous involvement should be considered candidates for wide surgical excision. It may be necessary in the pilosebaceous region to place skin grafts if the area removed is extensive. Margins should be free of disease and frozen sections may be of assistance in defining clear margins.

Patients who have recurrent disease after surgical or laser therapy may be candidates for topical 5% 5-fluorouracil applied twice daily. Caution should be observed when using this medication in young, sexually active women who are capable of reproduction, because of the potential for teratogenicity. Long-term use of 5% 5-fluorouracil will be required. In approximately 10 days after beginning 5% 5-fluorouracil application, the patient will begin to notice reddened, ulcerative skin on the vulva. At this point it is usually too painful to continue the applications; however, to effect maximum response, topical applications should be continued for several weeks. Most patients will be unable to accomplish this and it will be necessary to discontinue topical therapy. Patients at particular risk for recurrence are immunosuppressed patients. It may be advantageous in these patients to use prophylactic 5% 5-fluorouracil with application twice per week when healing has occurred after laser or excisional surgery. The efficacy of this approach, however, is not established.

Progressive Therapeutic Options

1. Wide, local excision for isolated, unicentric lesions for both diagnosis and therapy. Obtain an approximate 0.5-cm margin to document clear margins.
2. For large or multicentric disease, laser ablation to approximately 1 mm in nonpilosebaceous skin and local excision or laser ablation to 2.5 mm in pilosebaceous skin, with surrounding ablation giving a clear zone of approximately 1 cm peripheral to the intraepithelial neoplasia.
3. Wide excision of lesions in the pilosebaceous region that demonstrate deep skin appendage involvement on extensive preoperative histologic sampling.
4. For recurrent lesions, histologically proven to be noninvasive, consider topical 5% 5-fluorouracil twice daily. Advise that significant irritation will result from this topical therapy. The patient *must not conceive* on this regimen and must be advised of potential teratogenicity, if conception occurs.

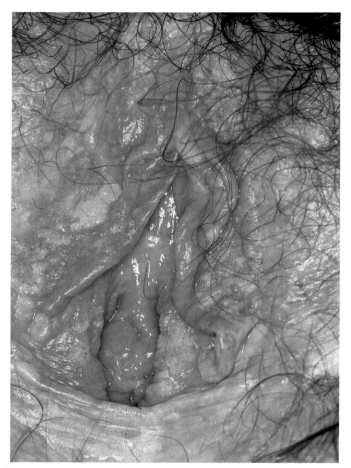

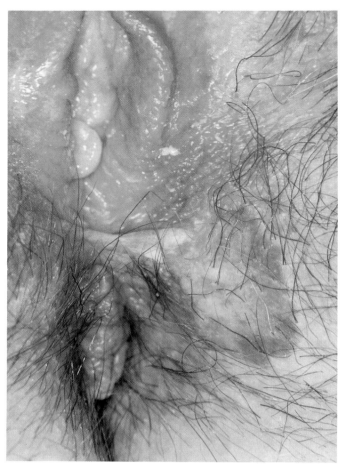

Figure 6.25. Diffuse plaques of white epithelium in a 25-year-old woman with history of two prior laser treatments. Biopsies demonstrated VIN 2 (polymerase-chain reaction was positive for HPV 16/18).

Figure 6.26. Hyperpigmented, localized lesion in an asymptomatic patient. Biopsy demonstrated VIN 2/3 and lesion was excised under general anesthesia with confirmation of diagnosis. Skin was undermined and closed with a permanent suture, which was removed 10 days later.

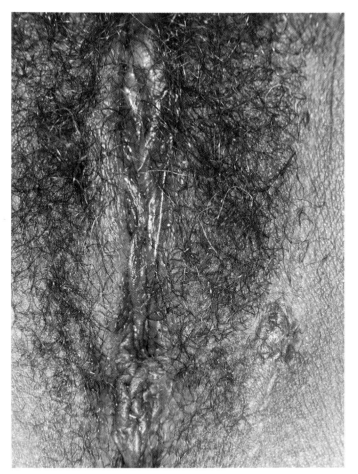

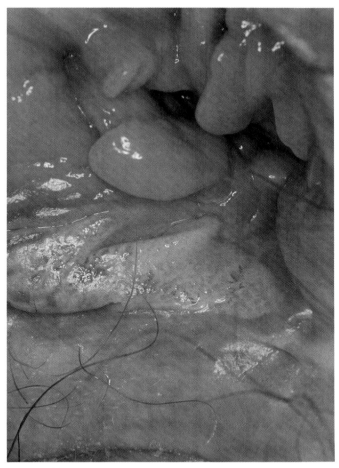

Figure 6.27. Hyperpigmented, solitary lesion in a woman who stated lesion had been present "since birth." Presumptive diagnosis was compound nevus; however, excisional biopsy demonstrated VIN 3.

Figure 6.28. Thickened white epithelium at introitus. Note prominent fissure. Excisional biopsy demonstrated VIN 3.

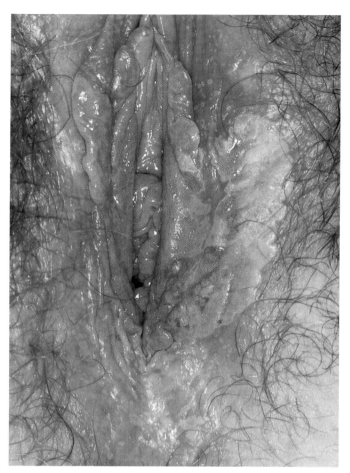

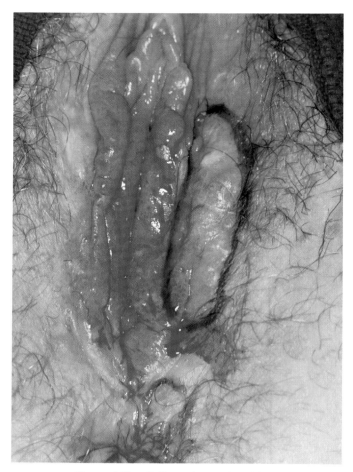

Figure 6.29. Left labial plaque demonstrating VIN 3 on biopsy. Plaque was excised under general anesthesia and surrounding skin was laser ablated to second and third surgical planes (Figure 6.31). Excised specimen demonstrated invasive squamous cell carcinoma (maximum depth of invasion 1.6 mm) (see Figures 6.30 and 6.31).

Figure 6.30. Delineated area of excision.

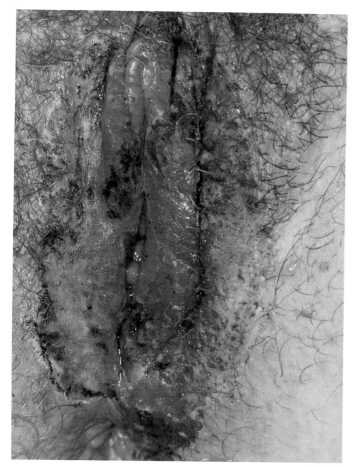

Figure 6.31. Excision has been approximated and surrounding VIN has been laser ablated.

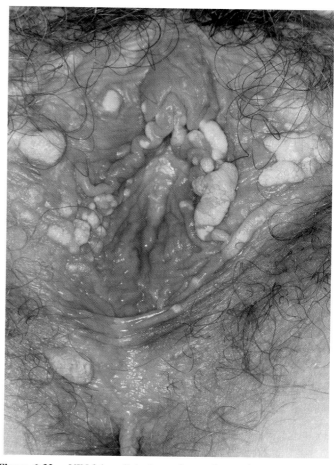

Figure 6.32. VIN 3 in a diabetic renal transplant patient taking Imuran (azothioprine), prednisone, cyclosporine, and insulin. Patient received excisional biopsy, laser ablation, 9 weeks of interferon injections, and 5% 5-fluorouracil topically, but VIN 3 persisted (see Figure 6.33).

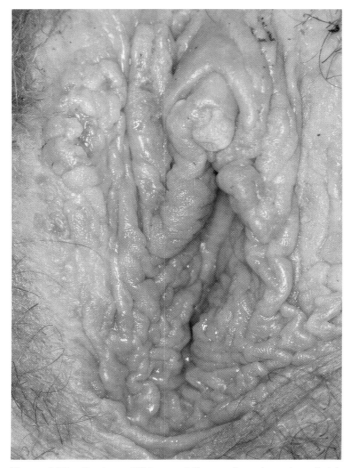

Figure 6.33. Persistent VIN, especially prominent in region of right labium majus (see Fig. 6.32).

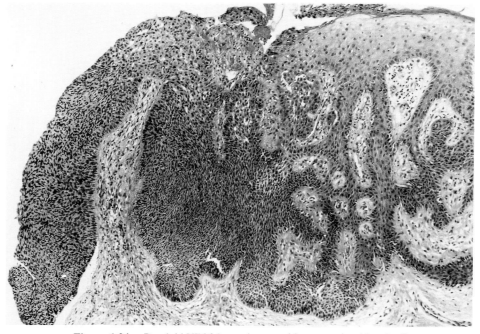

Figure 6.34. Basaloid VIN 3 is contiguous with an associated basal cell carcinoma.

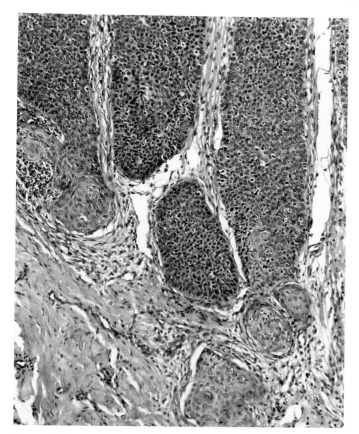

Figure 6.35. Basaloid VIN 3 with associated squamous cell carcinoma seen at the deep rete tips and in the dermis.

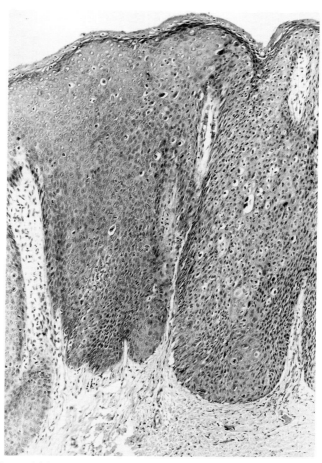

Figure 6.36. VIN 3, warty type. The epithelium has disorganized epithelial cell growth with lack of evidence of cellular maturation involving nearly the full thickness. The deeper rete ridges have a well-defined epidermal-dermal junction with a mild chronic inflammatory infiltrate in the superficial dermis.

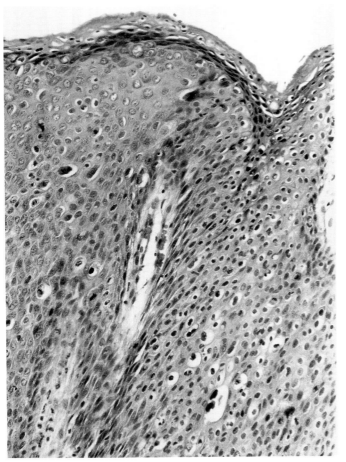

Figure 6.37. VIN, warty type. A higher magnification of Figure 6.34. The superficial keratinocytes have enlarged hyperchromatic nuclei with multinucleation and koilocytosis. Parakeratosis is present.

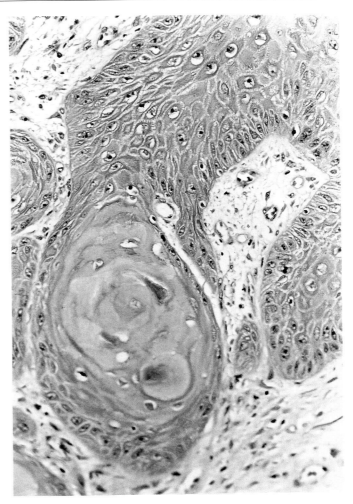

Figure 6.38. VIN 3, well-differentiated type, with squamous cell carcinoma. Within the tip of a rete ridge, keratinocytes with increased eosinophilic cytoplasm, dyskeratosis, and nuclear pleomorphism with prominent nucleoli are present within the parabasalar area.

7

TUMORS

BENIGN TUMOR ALGORITHM

TUMOR (Latin tumere: to swell):
a new growth of tissue, a neoplasm

Location	Presumed Diagnosis
Sulcus (labium minus/ labium majus)	Hidradenoma Papilliferum
Labium Majus	Acrochordon Granular cell Hemangioma Leiomyoma Lipoma
Mons, perineum	Endometriosis

Figure 7.1. Tumor algorithm.

Fibroepithelial Polyp (Acrochordon)

DEFINITION

A fibroepithelial polyp is a benign polypoid mass composed of a fibrovascular core and covered by stratified squamous epithelium that is keratinized.

CLINICAL PRESENTATION

An acrochordon is usually asymptomatic, noted by the patient only upon palpation or visual examination. Present for a number of years, rarely it may expand in size sufficiently to result in formation of a "giant acrochordon." Blood supply to the "giant acrochordon" may be compromised and ulceration may occur.

The diagnosis is suspected upon visual inspec-

tion. The polypoid structure appears fleshy and may feel like an empty sac. Smaller acrochordons may resemble an intradermal or dermal nevus. The soft consistency of the acrochordon assists in differentiating it from the typical firm condyloma, which may also appear as a polypoid vulvar lesion. Ultimately, the final diagnosis is dependent upon histologic confirmation.

MICROSCOPIC FINDINGS

Fibroepithelial polyps are found on hair-bearing skin of the vulva. They are soft and fleshy and may be pigmented. Their surface epithelium is keratinized squamous epithelium and may vary in appearance from thickened, acanthotic, and hyperkeratotic to flattened and thinned with a thin keratin layer. These polyps are of two distinct types, namely those that are predominantly epithelial and those that are primarily stromal. The stalk and cone of the polyp are composed of loosely bundled collagen with supporting vasculature. The stromal cells may exhibit nuclear pleomorphism and atypia but this is not common.

CLINICAL BEHAVIOR AND TREATMENT

The small asymptomatic acrochordon does not require excision unless concern exists about the diagnosis. Many patients will request removal because the acrochordon creates a sense of discomfort associated with clothing apparel. A laterally situated acrochordon may interfere with restrictive elastic bands on undergarments. The giant acrochordon will create obvious problems; the mere presence of a large lesion between the thighs may result in discomfort while walking. Excision may be accomplished in the office setting after placing a ligature around the base of the acrochordon. The base can be injected with a local anesthetic before placement of the ligature.

Progressive Therapeutic Options

1. No therapy is necessary for the acrochordon that has been present for years without symptoms.
2. Office excision of the symptomatic acrochordon for therapy and histologic confirmation of diagnosis is also indicated.

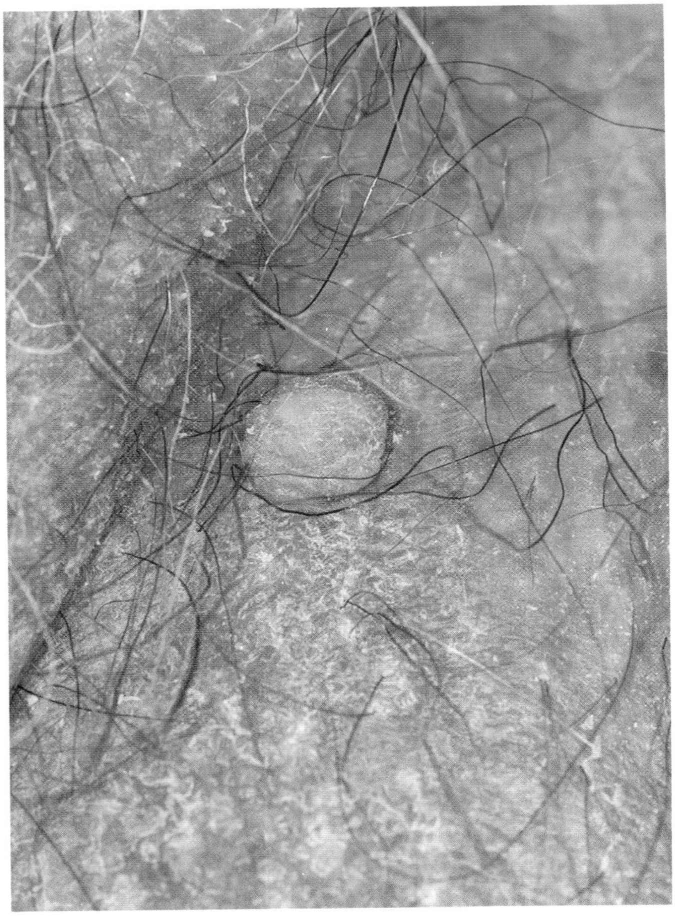

Figure 7.2. Fibroepithelial polyp (acrochordon) with typical papule appearance, similar to intradermal nevus. Excision confirmed diagnosis.

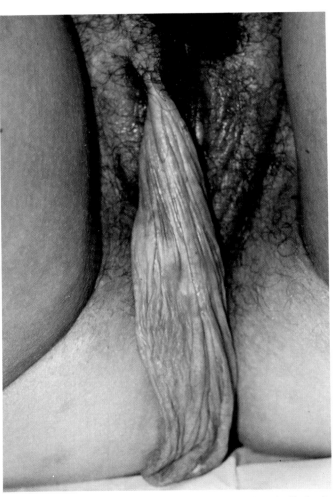

Figure 7.3. Giant acrochordon, which had increased markedly in size during pregnancy.

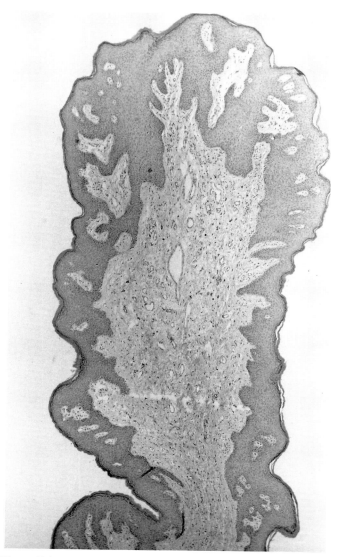

Figure 7.4. Fibroepithelial polyp. The epithelial surface is keratinized squamous epithelium. The epithelium is moderately thickened and acanthotic, especially in the distal tip of the polyp. A fibrovascular core, which has some thinly walled larger central vessels, supports the polyp.

Endometriosis

DEFINITION

Endometriosis is the ectopic implantation of endometrial glands and stroma.

GENERAL FEATURES

Endometriosis of the vulva is almost invariably secondary to implantation of fragments of endometrium in incisions such as episiotomies. It is a rare occurrence and is often enigmatic because episiotomy is a routine procedure performed with many, if not most, vaginal deliveries.

CLINICAL PRESENTATION

A patient with endometriosis of the vulva usually presents with cyclic enlargement and discomfort noted at the site of implantation. She will have had a history of a prior childbirth and an episiotomy, or will have a history of cesarean section (or hysterotomy) and will complain of suprapubic swelling and localized discomfort in the surgical incision. Although endometriosis of the vulva is usually a well-circumscribed lesion, endometriosis of the mons may be more diffuse and involve subcuticular adipose tissue and fascia.

MICROSCOPIC FINDINGS

The histopathologic features of endometriosis are as seen in other sites. Both endometrial glands and stroma are normally found, and hemosiderin-laden macrophages may be evident. The endometriosis may be within scar tissue, resulting in a firm, nodular, blue-black mass. In such cases, foreign body giant cells containing polarizable suture material are often found. Endometriosis may be primarily in the superficial dermis with a thinned overlying squamous epithelium. In such cases, cyst formation may occur within the endometriosis. The cyst contents are typically brown to black and slightly mucoid. Pregnant patients, or patients who have had progestin or antigonadotropin therapy, may have only a remaining endometrial stromal component, which may have decidual change. In such cases decidualized stromal cells and hemosiderin-laden macro-

phages are the only findings, and are considered consistent with endometriosis when identified.

ADJUNCTIVE STUDIES

If the patient complains of hematochezia and the endometriosis is in the perineum, then consideration should be given to direct visualization of the lower gastrointestinal tract to rule out transmural endometriosis. Similarly, urinary symptoms in patients with endometriosis should prompt endoscopic evaluation of the bladder.

DIFFERENTIAL DIAGNOSIS

A firm, indurated region of endometriosis may be difficult to differentiate from infiltrating carcinoma or a chronic infectious process. Superficial implants of endometriosis in the perineal body may be confused with an epidermal inclusion cyst or vestibular cyst.

CLINICAL BEHAVIOR AND TREATMENT

Endometriosis of the vulva is not a pharmacologic disease; it is a surgical disease, provided symptoms warrant removal. Small lesions of endometriosis may be removed in the clinic. Any suspicion of rectal mucosal involvement will require more extensive surgery, often necessitating sphincter repair and rectal wall repair. This is more easily accomplished after a bowel preparation and after appropriate anesthesia (general or regional). Endometriosis involving the mons usually will require significant resection in the operating room and any suspicion of bladder involvement should prompt appropriate preoperative assessment of bladder integrity. If endometriosis is extensive and surgical resection appears to have been suboptimal then gonadotropin-releasing hormone agonist therapy may be given monthly for 3–6 months postoperatively to enhance resorption of residual endometriosis.

Progressive Therapeutic Option

1. Excision for diagnosis and treatment is indicated.

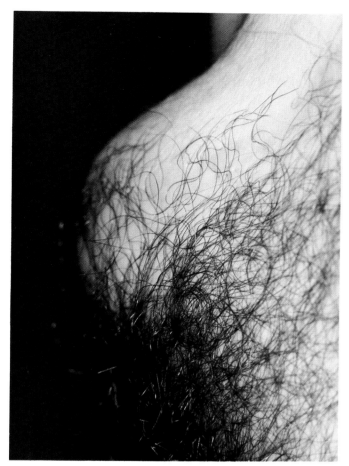

Figure 7.5. Endometrioma of the mons observed at site of prior hysterotomy for hematometra.

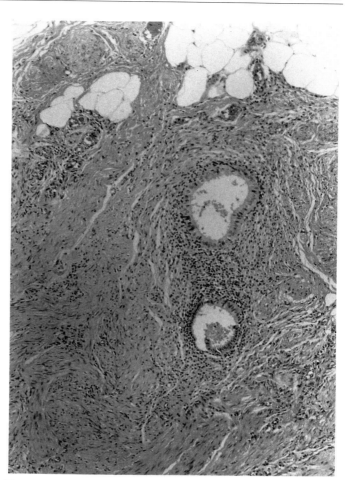

Figure 7.6. Endometriosis. Endometrial type glands and stroma are present.

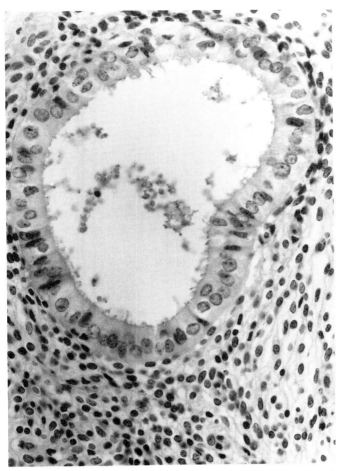

Figure 7.7. Endometriosis. Higher magnification demonstrating the tubal-endometrial–type epithelial cell lining and stromal cells.

Granular Cell Tumor

DEFINITION

Granular cell tumors are generally benign neoplasms considered to be of peripheral nerve sheath origin.

GENERAL FEATURES

Granular cell tumors may arise in children as well as adults and are most often seen in skin, subcutaneous tissue, and the tongue. They are more common in women than in men and blacks are more commonly affected than are whites.

CLINICAL PRESENTATION

The patient will typically present noting a nodular mass within the body of the labium majus. Multiple tumors may be palpated. The patient may complain of a similar lesion on the tongue.

On examination the tumor will be nontender and will be palpated within the labium majus or in the vicinity of the clitoris. Multiple lesions may be noted.

MICROSCOPIC FEATURES

Granular cell tumor in the vulva is associated with pseudoepitheliomatous hyperplasia of the overlying epithelium in approximately one-half of the cases and can mimic squamous cell carcinoma. An ulcerated surface may be found in some cases. The underlying granular cell tumor is composed of large cells with poorly defined cell borders with coarse, eosinophilic, granular cytoplasm. The nuclei are relatively uniform in size and shape and have coarse hyperchromatic chromatin. The tumor has poorly defined deep margins and may have an infiltrative appearance. Granular cell tumors are immunoreactive for S100 protein as well as myelin basic protein, reflecting their peripheral nerve sheath origin. They may contain carcinoembryonic antigen.

Locally aggressive and malignant granular cell tumors may occur on the vulva and can be recognized microscopically and clinically by their local extensive growth or metastasis. Distinctive microscopic features to distinguish malignant granular cell tumors from their benign counterpart are usually not present and the malignant or locally aggressive behavior may not be recognized until local recurrence is identified.

DIFFERENTIAL DIAGNOSIS

The differential diagnosis includes invasive squamous cell carcinoma, metastatic carcinoma, and xanthogranulomatous inflammation. Typically squamous cell carcinoma has an ulcerative or raised surface, somewhat irregular border. Granular cell tumors are not ulcerative. Although they are not encapsulated, they do not give the examiner the impression of a widely infiltrating lesion, which would be seen with carcinoma. Xanthogranulomata are most commonly seen in infants and newborns and are present as multiple yellow to yellow-brown papules or nodules. They may occur as solitary lesions in adults.

CLINICAL BEHAVIOR AND TREATMENT

Although granular cell tumors are almost invariably benign, metastatic malignant granular cell tumor has been described. Given the uncertainty of clinical diagnosis, the dictum to excise all firm nodules should be followed. Wide local excision should be accomplished under appropriate anesthesia. Usually the vulvar lesions can be removed in the office. Recurrences may be noted and these may be excised similarly. Observation of lesions on the tongue would warrant referral to otolaryngology or oral surgery for disposition.

Progressive Therapeutic Options

1. Wide local excision and submission for histologic diagnosis.
2. Periodic follow-up to confirm no recurrence.

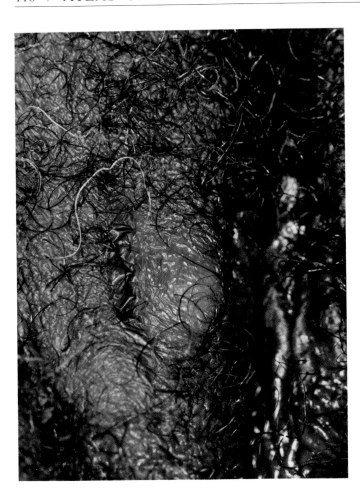

Figure 7.8. Granular cell tumor in the right labium majus. This had been removed 9 years before and had recurred recently in the same location.

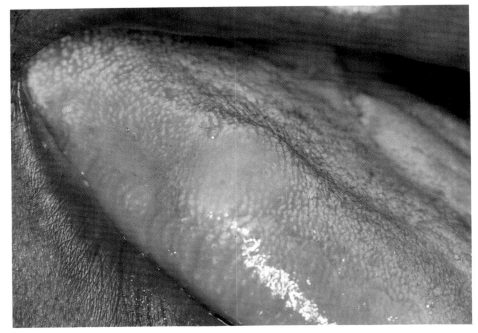

Figure 7.9. Granular cell tumors of the tongue in the same patient.

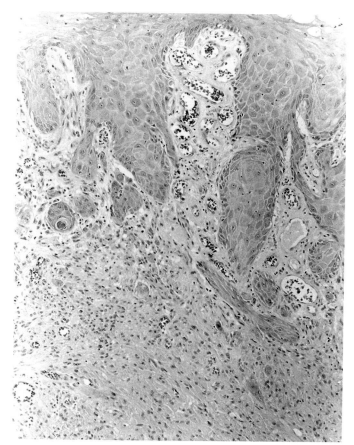

Figure 7.10. Granular cell tumor. In this case there is marked epithelial hyperplasia (pseudocarcinomatous hyperplasia) of the overlying epithelium. The granular cell tumor is present within the superficial dermis.

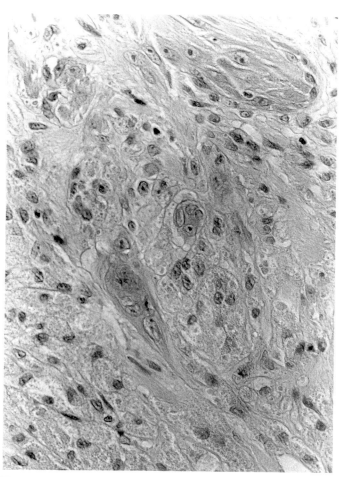

Figure 7.11. Granular cell tumor. Higher magnification of the adjacent figure illustrates the tumor in the dermis. The granular cells have uniform nuclei and prominent, coarsely granular cytoplasm.

Hemangioma

DEFINITION

A cavernous hemangioma is a vascular malformation resulting from dilated blood vessels with resultant formation of the vascular tumor deep within the dermis or subcutaneous tissues.

CLINICAL PRESENTATION

Cavernous hemangiomas usually present within the first few months of life and will frequently increase in size over the next several months. After a phase of rapid growth they may involute and regress or persist without subsequent growth. The infant with a cavernous hemangioma on the vulva may be presented for evaluation of the cosmetically disabling lesion. Rarely, the infant may be presented because of ulceration and bleeding of the vulvar hemangioma. The lesion may involve not only the vulva but the medial thighs and may extend deeply into the pelvic structures. Hemangiomas that persist may be a source of discomfort into adult life. Periodic thrombosis may result in significant pain.

The diagnosis of vulvar cavernous hemangioma is made by visual inspection. The appearance is diagnostic. For large hemangiomas, vascular phase magnetic resonance imaging (MRI) may define the depth of the hemangioma. The hemangioma may extend deeply into the pelvis and involve the pelvic side walls and perirectal spaces. This observation is of significance clinically for those patients who require therapy and for those patients who plan to conceive. A deep-seated cavernous hemangioma in the perivaginal wall and perirectal spaces may bleed significantly when exposed to the trauma of a vaginal delivery. Cesarean delivery would be more appropriate. Definition of hemangioma extent is also mandatory in patients for whom pelvic surgery, such as hysterectomy, is being contemplated. Alternatives to surgical therapy should be considered strongly when MRI demonstrates deep pelvic hemangioma extension.

MICROSCOPIC FINDINGS

Vulvar cavernous hemangiomas are generally best not biopsied and therefore are rarely encountered in surgical pathology. Microscopic features include variable-sized, endothelial-lined, blood-filled vascular spaces. In some cases, prominent smooth muscle may be seen about these vessels. The surrounding stroma may be fibrous and contain hemosiderin laden macrophages. Factor VIII antigen is demonstrable in the endothelial cells of hemangioma, but usually is absent in the endothelial cells of lymphangiomas. This finding, in addition to the presence of red cells in the vascular spaces of hemangiomas, is of value in discriminating hemangiomas from lymphangiomas.

CLINICAL BEHAVIOR AND TREATMENT

The typical asymptomatic cavernous hemangioma may be observed in infancy. Regression may occur and the hemangioma may resolve without the need for intervention. Persistent cavernous hemangiomas that are cosmetically disfiguring and are small, without evidence of deep involvement, may be excised when the child reaches an appropriate age for surgical intervention. Symptomatic lesions and those that may ulcerate may be managed with an argon laser or with the Nd:YAG laser. Augmentation of response may be accomplished by injecting the hemangioma with steroids.

Consideration should also be given to intervention in patients who develop the Kasabach-Merritt syndrome (thrombocytopenia and consumption coagulopathy secondary to a hemangioma). In such cases, the initial therapy should consist of oral prednisone; if no resolution is noted, then consideration should be given to laser or surgical intervention. Surgical intervention may be augmented with invasive radiographic embolization of the feeding vessels for the hemangioma. With diminution in blood flow surgical intervention then may be attempted. It should be remembered that surgical intervention for a deep vulvar cavernous hemangioma extending into the vaginal side walls and pelvis should not be attempted unless significant symptoms warrant the life-threatening risk of surgery.

Progressive Therapeutic Options

1. Observation and expectant waiting for resolution of the cavernous hemangioma of childhood.
2. Argon laser or Nd:YAG laser photocoagulation for ulcerative bleeding cavernous hemangiomas.
3. Surgical excision of small hemangiomas confined to the vulva.
4. Oral prednisone at 2–4 mg/kg/day for Kasabach-Merritt syndrome (see text).
5. Surgical resection after radiographic embolization for larger symptomatic vulvar hemangiomas. (Symptoms must warrant intervention.)
6. Avoidance of surgery for deep-seated cavernous hemangiomas involving the paravaginal and perirectal spaces.

NOTATION: Vascular phase MRI should be obtained when a cavernous hemangioma demonstrates evidence of deep extension (i.e., large lesions and lesions with concomitant leg involvement) to define pelvic extent of disease. Obtain the study preconceptually to assist in decisions concerning mode of delivery (cesarean section versus vaginal delivery). Obtain the study preoperatively when considering surgery for gynecologic disease and consider nonsurgical approaches or tailored surgical approaches when pelvic vascular involvement is noted.

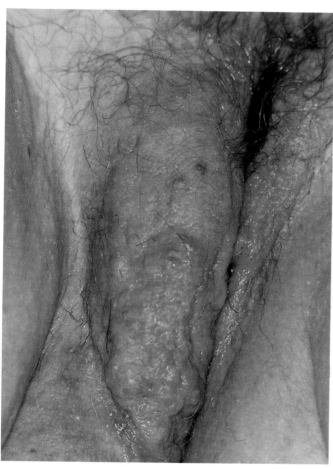

Figure 7.12. Variegated, nontender cavernous hemangioma of right labium majus. Vascular phase MRI demonstrated communication with deep pelvic hemangioma. No therapy was initiated.

Hidradenoma Papilliferum

DEFINITION

Hidradenoma papilliferum is a benign glandular tumor, believed to arise from specialized anogenital sweat glands.

GENERAL FEATURES

Found almost exclusively on the vulva in white women, it is extraordinarily rare for these tumors to be discovered in black women. Because the assumed derivation of these tumors is apocrine and black women have more apocrine glands in the vulvar region than do white women, the paucity of hidradenomas in the black population has raised questions concerning the presumed derivation of this tumor. This tumor may arise from specialized anogenital glands that are typically located in the interlabial sulci, a common location of vulvar hidradenomas.

MICROSCOPIC FINDINGS

On microscopic examination, hidradenoma papilliferum are composed of complex, glandular-type epithelium that are well defined and have discreet margins. The glandular epithelium may be papillary and cribriform in configuration. The epithelial cells typically have an underlying myoepithelial cell layer immediately above the basement memberane, which is immunoreactive for smooth muscle actin. Because of the complex structure of these neoplasms, they may mimic adenocarcinoma; however, there is typically no significant nuclear atypia. Myoepithelial cells are evident, and the process is well circumscribed. Adequately deep and complete excision is of great value in making the correct diagnosis. Occasionally, epithelial cell elements are found in the immediately adjacent stroma and are thought to represent trapped elements of the gland. Unlike normal sweat glands and tumors of sweat gland origin, hidradenoma papilliferum do not contain carcino-embryonic antigen, a finding that challenges this origin from typical apocrine glands.

CLINICAL PRESENTATION

The patient with hidradenoma papilliferum usually will present complaining of a small nodule discovered on vulvar self-examination. The nodule will be mobile and is typically located in the sulcus between the labium minus and labium majus. Occasionally these tumors may be found in the perineal tissue and they have been noted in distant sites such as the nipple and the eyelid. Rarely will the hidradenoma be tender. Occasionally these tumors may ulcerate and the patient may present complaining of pain and bleeding. Examination will demonstrate an ulcerated, mobile nodule in the usual location. The association of hidradenoma with adenocarcinoma is exceedingly rare.

A preliminary diagnosis of hidradenoma papilliferum may be made based upon the characteristic clinical picture. Confirmation of diagnosis requires excision and histopathologic examination.

CLINICAL BEHAVIOR AND TREATMENT

Excision is the therapeutic option for hidradenoma papilliferum. This may be accomplished in the office by infiltrating the area with lidocaine and excising the small nodule. This will allay the patient's concerns and result in confirmation of the presumed clinical diagnosis. Certainly the patient should be included in the decision to remove this benign tumor. If it has been present for several years and has been asymptomatic, then she may elect not to have it removed. The patient should understand that on rare occasion carcinoma has been noted to arise in a previous hidradenoma papilliferum.

Progressive Therapeutic Option

1. Simple excision.

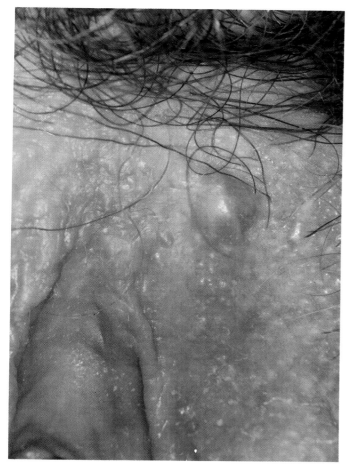

Figure 7.13. Asymptomatic hidradenoma. Note the location in the sulcus between the labium minus and majus.

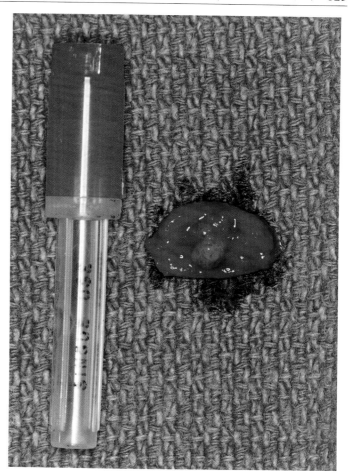

Figure 7.14. The hidradenoma after excision. Note the papillary projection within the cystic-appearing cavity.

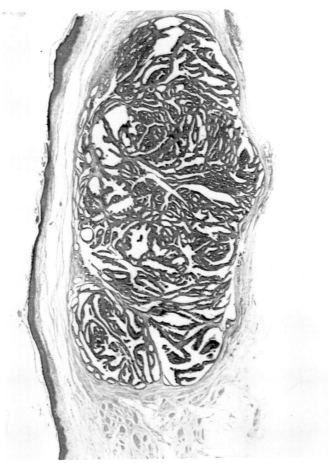

Figure 7.15. Papillary hidradenoma. Low magnification demonstrates the fully excised neoplasm, which is a complex, papillarylike neoplasm with a villoglandular pattern of growth. The tumor has a well-demarcated dermal junction and is not infiltrative.

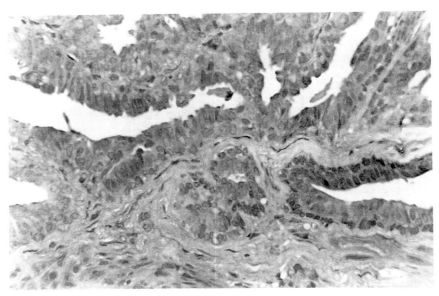

Figure 7.16. Papillary hidradenoma. Higher magnification demonstrates the myoepithelial cells underlying columnar secretory epithelium.

Leiomyoma

DEFINITION

Leiomyoma is a smooth muscle tumor of the vulva that may arise from smooth muscle in blood vessels, erectile tissue, and skin smooth muscle of the erector pili.

GENERAL FEATURES

Leiomyoma of the vulva is a relatively rare entity, unlike the more common leiomyoma of the uterus, although it represents the most common soft tissue tumor of the vulva.

CLINICAL PRESENTATION

Although these tumors rarely exceed 7 cm in diameter, it is more common for the patient to present with a smaller mass that is subcutaneous. The lesion typically will be in the labium majus and will be fairly mobile. If degeneration is present, the leiomyoma will appear soft and similar to a lipoma. Otherwise it will have the same firm consistency as noted when examining a leiomyoma of the uterus.

MICROSCOPIC FINDINGS

Vulvar leiomyomata are composed of smooth muscle cells arranged in complex interlacing and parallel fascicles. The cells have indiscrete cellular borders and contain eosinophilic cytoplasm, which is immunoreactive for actin, desmin, and myosin, characteristic of smooth muscle. The nuclei are relatively uniform and are oval or rounded. Mitosis are rare, under 5 per 10 high-power fields. Nuclear atypia, mitosis counts of 5 per 10 high-power fields or higher, and infiltration are characteristics of leiomyosarcoma. Epithelioid leiomyoma, with typical rounded smooth muscle cells resembling squamous cells, may occur in the vulva, and should be distinguished from squamous cell carcinoma. Vulvar rhabdomyoma may resemble leiomyoma; however, these tumors arise from striated muscle and contain myoglobin.

CLINICAL BEHAVIOR AND TREATMENT

As with a leiomyoma of the uterus, growth of the vulvar leiomyoma may be variable and it may increase in size with the passage of time. Given this tendency and given the inability to make a diagnosis without surgical pathology, treatment involves excision. After removal of the mass, malignancy can be ruled out by histologic evaluation.

Progressive Therapeutic Option

1. Surgical excision.

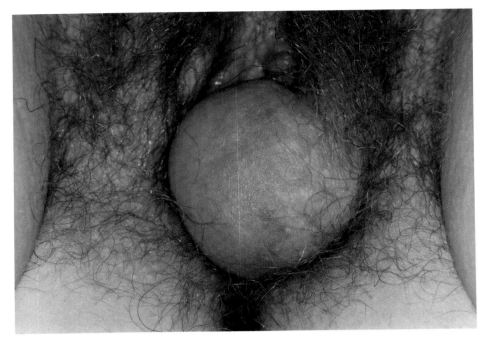

Figure 7.17. Leiomyoma of the vulva.

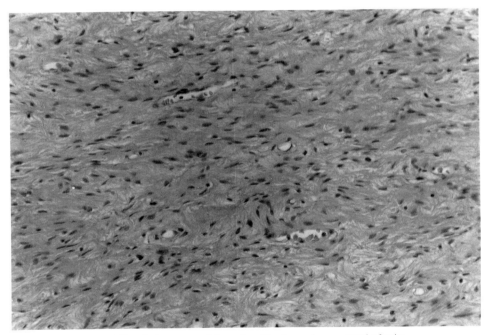

Figure 7.18. Leiomyoma of the vulva. The tumor is composed of spindle-shaped smooth muscle cells arranged in interlacing bundles. The nuclei are in the center of the cell on cross-section and are uniform in size and shape. Rare mitotic figures may be found.

Lipoma

DEFINITION

A lipoma is a benign tumor occurring on the vulva and is composed primarily of fat cells (adipocytes).

CLINICAL PRESENTATION

The patient with a symptomatic lipoma will usually present complaining of a mass on the vulva in the region of the labium majus. Frequently this mass will have been present for a number of years, but increase in size will prompt concern and desire for further evaluation.

The diagnosis is suspected when a soft, well-circumscribed mass is palpated within the body of the labium majus. The overlying skin is normal in appearance.

MICROSCOPIC FINDINGS

Lipomas may be highly variable in their relation to the surface epithelium. They may vary from deep in a vulvar fat pad to pedunculated, forming a broad-based, soft, polypoid mass. The tumor is composed of adipocytes with a fibrovascular connective tissue element. When the fibrous component is prominent, the term fibrolipoma is preferred. The adipocytes are immunoreactive for S100 and this may be of value in discriminating the adipocytes from adjacent fibrous tissue or when fibroma, hemangioma, or leiomyoma are within the differential diagnosis.

DIFFERENTIAL DIAGNOSIS

The differential diagnosis includes hemangioma, fibroma, leiomyoma, Bartholin's cyst and canal of Nuck cyst. A hemangioma will have a characteristic purple-red hue secondary to dilated vascular spaces. Leiomyomas and fibromas will be more solid upon palpation. The anatomic location of a Bartholin's cyst would assist in differentiating this from a lipoma. A canal of Nuck cyst will be soft and compressible, and may increase in size with increased intraabdominal pressure. Final diagnosis of lipoma is based on histologic examination.

CLINICAL BEHAVIOR AND TREATMENT

Small lipomas may be removed in the office under local anesthesia; however, most lipomas will require excision in the operating room. If redundant skin is noted an elliptical excision of overlying skin may result in a more acceptable cosmetic result when the distended epithelium is reapproximated after removal of the lipoma. Bleeding is rarely a problem and usually can be controlled with electrocautery and minimal ligature placement. Occasionally, a lipoma will dissect deeply into the paravaginal and pararectal tissues, requiring extensive resection.

Progressive Therapeutic Option

1. Excision.

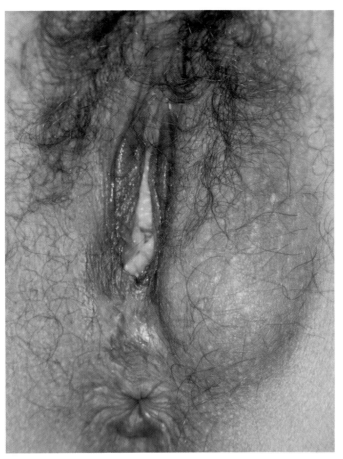

Figure 7.19. Seven-centimeter painful lipoma present for 3 years.

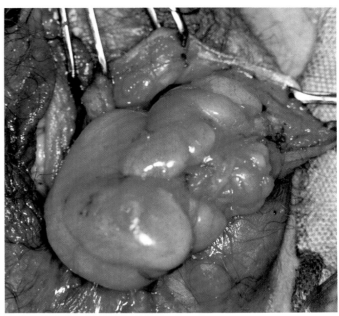

Figure 7.20. Gross appearance of excised lipoma of Figure 7.19.

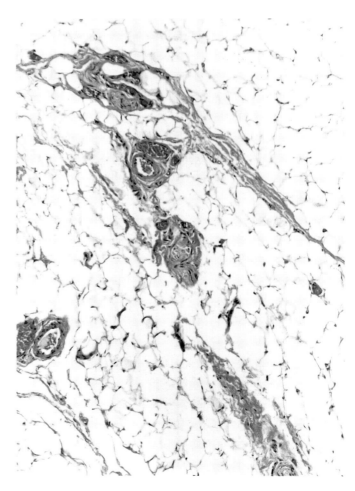

Figure 7.21. Lipoma of the vulva. The tumor is composed of benign-appearing adopocytes with intervening fibrous tissue. No nuclear pleomorphism or mitosis are present.

8

ULCERS

ULCER ALGORITHM

ULCER (Latin ulcus; Greek helkosis: wound): a transcutaneous (epidermis and dermis) defect

Presumed Diagnosis	Confirmation
AIDS	Western Blot (HIV)
Behçet's disease	Histology
Carcinoma	Histology
Chancroid	Culture (H. ducreyi)
Crohn's disease	Histology
Decubitus	Histology
Herpes	Culture (HSV)
Hidradenitis	Histology
Lymphogranuloma	Serology (Chlamydia)
Pemphigoid	Histology
Syphilis	Dark-field/serology (VDRL)
Systemic lupus erythematosus	Serology (antinuclear antibody)

Figure 8.1. Ulcer algorithm. Because of the overlap in symptoms and findings, no clinically useful algorithm to arrive at a presumed diagnosis is attempted. The algorithm deals only with confirmation of the diagnosis.

AIDS

DEFINITION

The acquired immunodeficiency syndrome (AIDS) is a consequence of infestation of helper lymphocytes with the retrovirus human immunodeficiency virus (HIV), resulting in failure of the host immune defense system and ultimately death as a consequence of the failure of the body's defense mechanisms.

CLINICAL PRESENTATION

Vulvar disease may be a primary presenting complaint in HIV infected patients whose HIV status is unknown. More commonly ulcerative disease discovered on the vulva is observed in patients who are known to be seropositive for HIV. The ulcers are frequently multiple and may involve the perianal, vulvar, and vaginal surfaces. They are frequently painful and may or may not demonstrate evidence of superimposed infection. Although usually the patient's HIV status is known, it must be remembered that these patients may have no other clinical stigmata of AIDS and therefore may present complaining solely of vulvar and perianal ulceration. A high clinical index of suspicion must be maintained.

The diagnosis is made by exclusion. Given the inability to differentiate vulvar ulceration purely on clinical criteria, it is necessary to obtain assays for those agents that commonly cause vulvar ulceration. Ulcers should be cultured for herpesvirus. Dark-field or immunofluorescent examination should be accomplished to evaluate for *Treponema pallidum*. Serologic studies specific for syphilis also should be obtained. Serology for *Chlamydia trachomatis* as the etiologic agent in lymphogranuloma venereum should be obtained. Cultures for *Hemophilus ducreyi*, the etiologic organism in chancroid, should be considered. If the HIV status of the patient is not known, then she should be counseled to obtain an HIV assay. If all assays return negative and the HIV assay is positive, then the presumptive diagnosis of primary HIV-induced vulvar ulceration may be made. Biopsy of the ulceration may be accomplished to assist in the diagnosis, but nonspecific inflammation will be observed typically.

MICROSCOPIC FINDINGS

Kaposi's sarcoma may involve the vulva in women with AIDS, but the lesions are usually multiple and found in other cutaneous sites. The lesions of Kaposi's sarcoma evolve over time from a patch to a plaque to a nodular lesion.

The microscopic feature in the patch phase includes a vascular neoplasm composed of thin-walled, irregularly shaped vessels with poorly defined margins that are peripherally separated by dermal collagen. Mononuclear inflammatory cells, consisting predominately of lymphocytes and plasma cells, are found within the interstitial tissues and perivascular spaces.

As the lesion develops to a plaque and then nodular mass, the vessels become more numerous and their irregular shape becomes more extreme. Surrounding the angulated and slitlike vascular spaces, atypical spindle cells are evident, that, in the nodular stage are a prominent feature and form a spindle-cell neoplasm with atypical spindle cells. Those tumors are poorly demarcated and highly vascular, and have infiltrative margins.

The main differential diagnosis is bacillary (epithelioid) angiomatosis, which is diagnosed by identifying the bacteria, *Rochalimaea henselae*. This bacterial rod can be identified on silver stain, such as Walthin-Starry stain. When the Kaposi's sarcoma is relatively solid other spindle-cell neoplasms, including angiosarcoma and fibrous histiocytoma, may be considered in the differential diagnosis.

The epithelioid neoplastic cells of angiosarcoma contain multilocular cytoplasmic vacuoles. Angiosarcomas are typically more vascular than Kaposi's sarcoma. Fibrohistiocytomas are immunoreactive for α_1-antitrypsin, α_1-antichymotrypsin. They have a storiform arrangement of the spindled neoplastic cells and lack the blood-filled, irregular vascular spaces of Kaposi's sarcoma.

CLINICAL BEHAVIOR AND TREATMENT

Initiation of zidovudine at 100 mg orally every 4 hours five times per day or 200 mg every 8 hours may be effective in controlling the vulvar ulcerations induced by HIV. Ulcerations may also occur in the mouths of patients who are HIV positive and may be a primary manifestation of HIV. These ulcerations often do not heal in response to numerous pharmacologic agents such as acyclovir, ketoconazole, or topical steroids. Moderately high doses of oral steroids have been efficacious in resolving these oral ulcerations. Dosages of prednisone consist of 40 mg per day for 1 week, followed by 20 mg of prednisone per day for the second week. This regimen may be considered in a patient with vulvar ulceration secondary to HIV in whom all appropriate evaluations have ruled out secondary causes for the ulcerations and in whom zidovudine has not effected a response.

Progressive Therapeutic Options

1. After confirmation of HIV seropositivity and negative assessment for secondary etiologies, zidovudine 100 mg orally every 4 hours five times per day or 200 mg every 8 hours.
2. Consider systemic steroid intervention with oral prednisone, 40 mg per day for 1 week, followed by 20 mg per day for 1 week.

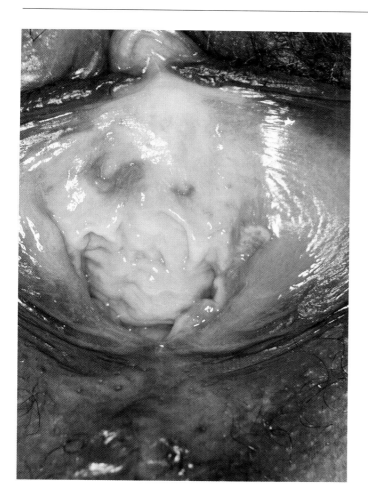

Figure 8.2. Multiple vestibular ulcerations in patient with erosive vaginitis and known AIDS. Complete microbiologic and serologic evaluation was negative and biopsy demonstrated inflammation.

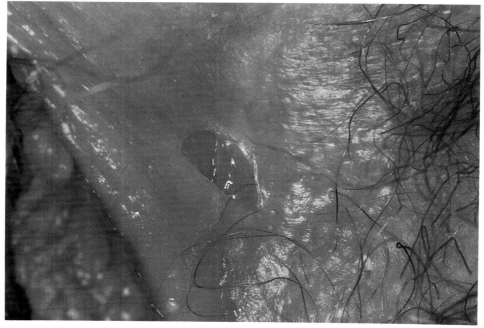

Figure 8.3. Deep "punched-out" ulcer in AIDS patient with negative microbiologic and serologic evaluation (dark-field, VDRL, Gram stain, *Chlamydia* assay, and HSV culture). Biopsy demonstrated inflammation.

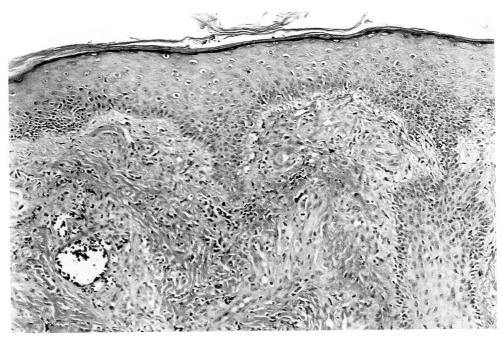

Figure 8.4. Kaposi's sarcoma. At low magnification the spindled-cell neoplasm is evident within the superficial dermis. Some unusual prominent superficial vessels are also present. The overlying epithelium is abutted by the neoplastic process.

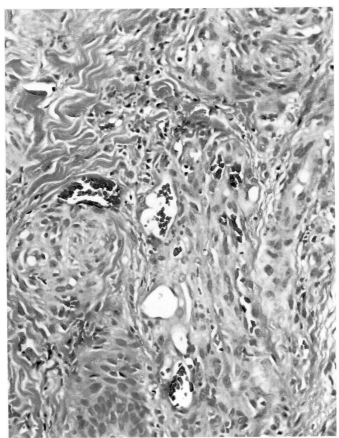

Figure 8.5. Kaposi's sarcoma. A higher magnification of the adjacent figure demonstrates the multiple small, blood-filled vessels and spindled cells enmeshed within the dermal collagen.

Behçet's Disease (Syndrome)

DEFINITION

Behçet's syndrome consists of the clinical triad of oral ulcers, genital ulcers, and ophthalmologic inflammation.

GENERAL FEATURES

Behçet's disease is a multisystem inflammatory disease resulting from a primary vasculitis. The etiology is unknown, although genetic and immunologic features have been observed. The disease is most common in the Orient, particularly Japan and in Mediterranean countries, particularly Turkey. A much lower prevalence is noted in patients of Northern-European extraction. There is also the observation that the HLA-B51 antigen has a higher prevalence in patients with Behçet's syndrome.

CLINICAL PRESENTATION

Patients will most commonly present with multiple, painful, aphthous ulcers. Numerous systems may be involved with clinical manifestations ranging from mild discomfort because of the ulceration to life-threatening ischemia secondary to the underlying vasculitis and associated thrombophlebitis. Systems involved may include eyes, joints, central nervous system, gastrointestinal tract, and the skin and mucosal surfaces. Progressive eye disease may eventuate in blindness; however, not all cases have ocular changes. Central nervous system involvement may manifest itself as headaches that may progress to seizures related to encephalopathy. Gastrointestinal disease with colitis may progress to perforation of the colon eventuating in sepsis and death.

Patients who present to the gynecologist for evaluation will usually present complaining of painful vulvar ulcerations which preclude intercourse. The ulcers may be deep and fenestration of the labia as well as gangrene of the labia may occur. The ulcers will be quite tender to the touch. Examination of the patient's buccal mucosa will frequently demonstrate multiple similar ulcerations.

Diagnosis of Behçet's disease requires adherence to the international diagnostic criteria for Behçet's disease. In addition to the observation of oral ulcerations, two additional clinical observations must be made from the following:

1. recurrent genital ulcerations,
2. eye lesions (uveitis, retinal vasculitis),
3. dermatologic lesions (erythema nodosum, papular-pustular lesions or acneiform lesions),

4. a positive pathergy test (intradermal injection of sterile water resulting in formation of a papule or pustule 48 hours later).

MICROSCOPIC FINDINGS

The key histologic feature is necrotizing arteritis, which is typically associated with endothelial cell swelling that may occlude arterial lumens. Associated venous thrombosis is also commonly observed. A chronic perivascular inflammatory infiltrate is typically present that can extend into the vascular wall of the involved vessels and be associated with homogenization of the media of the involved vessels.

ADJUNCTIVE STUDIES

The vulvar ulcerations should be cultured for herpesvirus. Immunofluorescent or dark-field examination should be performed to rule out syphilis. Appropriate serologic studies (Venereal Disease Research Laboratory [VDRL] or Rapid Plasma Reagin [RPR]) should be obtained as well. The patient should be counseled for, and receive, screening for HIV. Likewise, chlamydial serology should be obtained to assess for the possibility of lymphogranuloma venereum.

DIFFERENTIAL DIAGNOSIS

The diagnosis of Behçet's disease must be suspected when vulvar ulcerations are observed. Other diseases to be included in this differential are herpes, syphilis, pemphigoid, pemphigus, Crohn's disease, lymphogranuloma venereum, and AIDS. Exclusion of Crohn's disease may be difficult. Patients with Crohn's disease typically do not have oral ulcerations. Crohn's disease of the vulva is usually more lateral, involving the skin lateral to the labia majora, resulting in deep-seated, knifelike ulcerations between the labia majora and the medial thighs. Behçet's disease tends to involve the more medial aspects of the vulva. Biopsy may be necessary to differentiate the two conditions because both may involve the bowel. Crohn's disease is a granulomatous disease, whereas Behçet's disease is primarily a vasculitis. Rarely, both diseases may exist in the same patient. Pemphigus and cicatricial pemphigoid may involve the oral mucosa and eventuate in ulcers. To differentiate these conditions from Behçet's will require biopsy of vulvar skin and submission for direct immunofluorescent studies. Indirect immunofluorescent studies using the patient's serum may also be of assistance in evaluating for these two conditions. The ultimate diagnosis of

Behçet's syndrome will require the exclusion of these causes of vulvar ulcerations.

CLINICAL BEHAVIOR AND TREATMENT

The ulcerations typically recur and are usually associated with oral ulcers. Management of vulvar Behçet's disease is accomplished primarily with application of topical steroids. Moderate-strength steroids such as betamethasone valerate 0.1% applied twice daily for 1–2 weeks may result in alleviation of the inflammatory response. To control pain this may be augmented with topical applications of 2% viscous lidocaine or 5% Xylocaine ointment. Vigorous local hygiene consisting of sitz baths may also be comforting. If this fails to alleviate discomfort, then perilesional injections of triamcinolone acetonide (Kenalog-10) may be accomplished, resulting in wheal formation under the lesion. Although the use of birth control pills has been advocated to control vulvar disease, their use should be carefully considered, especially if patients note symptoms in other organ systems. Birth control pills are relatively contraindicated in patients with vascular disease. Anecdotal reports of the efficacy of acyclovir in managing vulvar Behçet's disease may support a clinical trial; however, there is no known association between herpesvirus and Behçet's disease. With disabling genital ulceration it may be necessary to initiate systemic steroids in dosages of 20–60 mg/day with subsequent tapering after disease activity is reversed. Failure of systemic steroids to control the disease may require the initiation of immunosuppressant therapy. Azathioprine (Imuran) at 1–2 mg/kg/day may result in a significant clinical response and the ability to diminish steroid dosaging. Careful monitoring should be accomplished when using immunosuppressant therapy with azathioprine (complete blood cell count, liver function tests, amylase and lipase levels). This medication should be used by those familar with its use and potential toxicity. Immunosuppressant therapy should be initiated only to control severe disease. Cyclosporine is an immunosuppressant that may be of benefit in patients who are unable to tolerate azathriopine; however, disease activity must be severe to warrant initiation. Long-term concerns include the association between cyclosporine and renal dysfunction as well as the development of neoplasm. Lastly, colchicine at 1.5 mg/day may be considered, although it seems to be most effective in managing erythema nodosum observed with Behçet's disease. The role of colchicine in managing vulvar ulcerations is not defined.

Progressive Therapeutic Options

1. Meticulous vulvar hygiene with sitz baths.
2. Topical betamethasone valerate 0.1% ointment twice daily for 2 weeks and then taper use.
3. Topical therapy with viscous lidocaine gel 2% or 5% Xylocaine ointment.
4. Perilesional injection of triamcinolone acetonide (Kenalog-10), creating a wheal under the ulcer.
5. Consider a trial of acyclovir 200 mg orally 5 times per day.
6. Consider a trial of estrogen-containing oral contraceptive if no evidence of multisystem vasculitis is present.
7. Consider a trial of colchicine 1.5 mg orally per day, especially if erythema nodosum is present.
8. For severe disease unresponsive to previous interventions, initiate oral prednisone at 20–60 mg/day and begin to taper after clinical response is noted.
9. For significant disease unresponsive to systemic steroid therapy, consider azathioprine (Imuran) starting at 1–2 mg/kg/day with subsequent increase in dosage to 2.5 mg/kg/day if no untoward toxicity noted (careful monitoring of complete blood cell count, liver function tests, lipase, amylase). With severe disease dose may be started at 2.5 mg/kg/day.
10. For patients unresponsive to azathioprine consider cyclosporine at 3–5 mg/kg/day with careful monitoring of blood parameters (complete blood cell count, liver function tests, cholesterol, triglyceride, electrolytes, urea nitrogen, creatine, creatinine clearance). Patients should be counseled extensively about the concern for renal dysfunction and potential development of extragenital neoplasia.

NOTATION: Immunosuppressant therapy should be used only by those familiar with its dosaging and side effects.

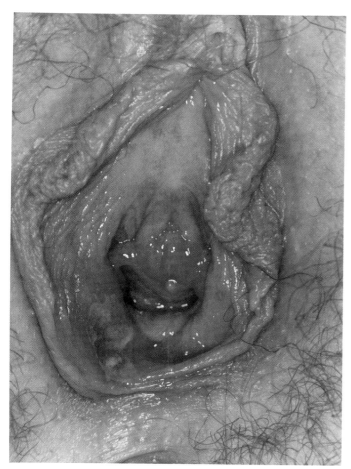

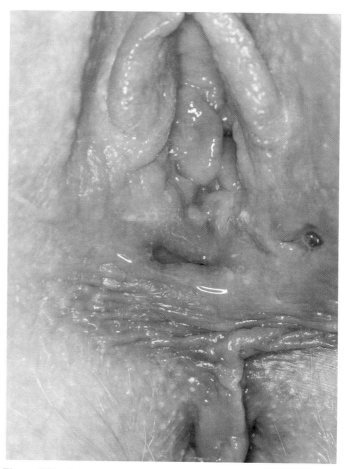

Figure 8.6. Painful ulcer in a patient with oral ulcerations and episodes of abdominal pain. Biopsy demonstrated vasculitis consistent with Behçet's disease. Evaluation (serologic and microbiologic) for other potential pathogens was negative. Acyclovir therapy resulted in resolution of ulcer and decreased frequency of oral ulcerations.

Figure 8.7. Deeply invasive ulcers (2 cm) in a patient with aphthous oral lesions and inflammatory bowel disease. Biopsy demonstrated vasculitis consistent with Behçet's disease. Therapy was initiated with prednisone and azthioprine (Imuran).

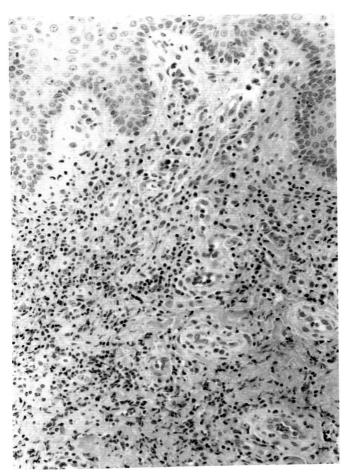

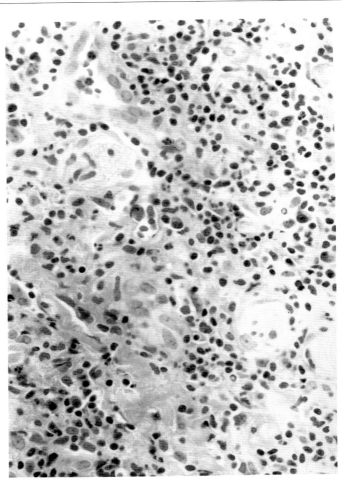

Figure 8.8. Behçet's disease. The severe inflammatory infiltrate predominantly consists of lymphocytes with some plasma cells, granulocytes, and eosinophils. Several vessels have microthrombi.

Figure 8.9. Behçet's disease. The overlying epithelium is lost in this deep biopsy from an ulcerated area. There is marked deep inflammatory infiltrate that is predominantly perivascular.

Chancroid

DEFINITION

A sexually transmitted disease caused by the organism *Haemophilus ducreyi*.

GENERAL FEATURES

Chancroid is a disease primarily of the tropics and subtropics, commonly observed in areas of prostitution. The disease is rarely seen in industrialized nations. Small epidemics have been noted in the United States, especially the south and southeastern United States. The disease more commonly affects men than women. There is a frequent association with HIV seropositivity.

The organism *H. ducreyi* is a Gram-negative, facultative, anaerobic bacillus that tends to exhibit streptobacillary chaining on Gram stain and culture.

CLINICAL PRESENTATION

After an initial incubation period of 3–5 days, papules will arise on the vulva in the region of the labia, forchette, and vestibule. Rarely, lesions may also be noted in the vagina and on the cervix. The papules will become pustular and ulcerate. The subsequent ulcers will enlarge and often have irregular borders that are somewhat undermined and surrounded by a red halo. There will be minimal to no induration and hence the term soft chancre is often used to describe the ulcer associated with *H. ducreyi*. The surface of the ulcer may appear grayish, especially if superinfection is present. Autoinoculation is common and various stages of development will be seen in the same patient (papules, pustules, and ulcers). The ulcers are usually tender. They may be present for weeks and months in the woman before symptoms become bothersome and prompt medical care. Ulcerations in the vagina and cervix may be asymptomatic. Unilateral or bilateral lymphadenopathy develops within 1–2 weeks and with progression of the disease, a bubo develops. Rupture results in formation of chronic draining inguinal sinuses. Similarly, ulcerations on the vulva that remain untreated may form chronic draining sinus tracts.

MICROSCOPIC FEATURES

H. ducreyi is the cause of chancroid and is a nonmotile, Gram-negative bacteria that can be cultured on selective agar medium and that, in culture, forms parallel chains and paired groups of bacteria. Culture identification is essential for definitive diagnosis.

The histologic features consist of a superficial and deep chronic granulomatous inflammatory infiltrate predominately composed of lymphocytes and plasma cells.

DIFFERENTIAL DIAGNOSIS

The two primary diseases that may be confused with chancroid involve ulcerations due to herpes simplex virus and ulcerations secondary to *T. pallidum* (syphilis).

It may be extremely difficult to differentiate herpetic lesions from those due to *H. ducreyi*. Herpetic lesions tend to be more painful and are associated with systemic manifestations when presenting as a primary infection. Herpetic lesions do not typically evolve through a papular-pustular state, but more commonly present as vesicles that subsequently ulcerate. Urinary symptoms are commonly noted with primary herpetic infections. Differentiation between the two conditions requires isolation of herpes simplex by culture or demonstration of herpesvirus cytologic findings on Tzanck smear.

Differentiation between chancroid and syphilis is relatively less complicated. Syphilitic chancres typically are not multiple unless autoinoculation has resulted in "kissing" lesions. The chancre of syphilis is nontender and is somewhat indurated (the hard ulcer). Syphilitic chancres have less tendency to have a grayish, "dirty" base. Diagnosis of syphilis is made by dark-field examination and sequential serology.

Primary HIV ulcerations should be considered in the differential diagnosis. These ulcers may be deeply invasive, demonstrating varying degrees of tenderness. The HIV-positive patient with vulvar ulcerations should be evaluated for all infectious causes of such ulcerations before designating the ulcerations as primarily induced by HIV. Such patients are at risk for chancroid, herpes, and syphilis.

Ultimately, the diagnosis of *H. ducreyi*-induced ulceration is based upon Gram-stain demonstration of coccobacillary chaining and culture isolation of *H. ducreyi*. Culture isolation requires selective media (gonococcal agar base and Mueller-Hinton agar base with Vancomycin), incubated at 33°C in CO_2 in a humid atmosphere. Most laboratories do not have culture capabilities for this organism and often superinfection of the vulvar ulcerations results in contamination with other organisms, making Gram-stain diagnosis impossible. In such cases a presumptive diagnosis of exclusion based upon the clinical presentation must be made and appropriate assays/cultures obtained for those conditions considered in the differential diagnosis (herpes, syphilis, HIV).

CLINICAL BEHAVIOR AND TREATMENT

Left untreated, chancroid may persist in women for several months, resulting in scarring, fistulae, and draining inguinal abscesses. Rarely, if remission occurs without treatment, relapse may be noted at the site of the original infection. With initiation of treatment there should be prompt resolution of the vulvar ulcerations, if the appropriate diagnosis has been made, and if antibiotic resistance is not problematic. Initial therapy should consist of oral administration of erythromycin 500 mg 4 times a day for 7 days. Alternative regimens include ceftriaxone 250 mg intramuscularly for one dose or azithromycin 1 g orally for one dose. For those patients allergic to these regimens, ciprofloxacin 500 mg may be administered orally twice daily for 3 days, provided the patient is not pregnant. Ciprofloxacin is contraindicated in pregnancy.

For patients with suppurating inguinal adenopathy, assistance may be obtained via needle aspiration of the bubo under local anesthesia. The needle should enter the abscess through normal skin, lateral and superior to the abscess. If there is reaccumulation of pus within the bubo, a second needle aspiration may be necessary. The bubo does not require surgical drainage, aspiration is sufficient.

Appropriate HIV screening is indicated in all patients with a diagnosis of chancroid, and appropriate counseling should be given.

Progressive Therapeutic Options

1. Erythromycin 500 mg orally four times a day for 7 days (or) ceftriaxone 250 mg intramuscularly once (or) azithromycin 1 g orally once (or) ciprofloxacin 500 mg orally twice daily for 3 days. (Ceftriaxone and azithromycin are less effective as single-dose therapy in HIV-infected patients.)
2. Needle aspiration superiorly and laterally through noninfected skin to drain an inguinal bubo.

NOTATION: Obtain an HIV assay after appropriate counseling of all patients with vulvar ulcerations.

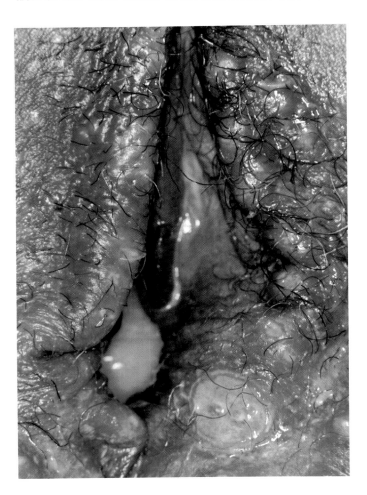

Figure 8.10. Multiple ulcerated papules and ulcers in various stages of development. These lesions have been present for approximately 2–3 weeks in a patient who had intercourse 4 weeks before presentation. The lesions were extremely tender. Herpes culture was negative. VDRL was nonreactive and Gram stain demonstrated nonspecific findings. HIV screen was negative.

Decubitus Ulcer

DEFINITION

A decubitus ulcer is destruction of skin and underlying tissues secondary to pressure necrosis.

GENERAL FEATURES

A vulvar decubitus ulcer is most commonly seen in paralyzed patients who do not use adequate padding to prevent necrosis of skin and underlying tissues resulting from pressure against the bony pelvis.

CLINICAL PRESENTATION

The paralyzed patient with a decubitus ulcer will not present until secondary infection has induced a localized process resulting in a significant discharge or until an ulcer is palpated on self-examination. The ulcer will overlie a bony prominence and will on occasion be sufficiently deep to expose the bone. In such instances the risk of osteitis exists. The most common locations of the ulcers are under the pubic rami (occurring when a patient sits on the arm of a wheelchair for prolonged periods of time), or just above the ischial tuberosities (occurring when maximum pressure is exerted on the buttocks when seated).

MICROSCOPIC FINDINGS

Decubitus ulcers are generally not biopsied and are usually recognized by their distinctive locations in the setting of the bed-ridden, or wheelchair-confined patient. The histopathologic features are nonspecific and the depth of ulceration is highly variable. In all cases, the epithelium is lost and the underlying dermis has a chronic inflammatory infiltrate without evidence of vasculitis. Organisms may be identified on silver or Brown and Brenn stains, but are confined to the surface of the ulcer.

ADJUNCTIVE STUDIES

In the typical case no adjunctive studies are necessary and often biopsy is unnecessary, given the patient's history and the location of the ulcer.

DIFFERENTIAL DIAGNOSIS

All etiologies of vulvar ulcerations may be considered in the differential diagnosis, but the typical location of the ulcerations over the ischial tuberosities or just under the pubic rami within the vestibule of the vulva usually will not warrant further studies. Biopsy will certainly exclude invasive squamous cell carcinoma; appropriate cultures assist in evaluating for herpesvirus; dark-field examination and serology will rule out syphilis.

CLINICAL BEHAVIOR AND TREATMENT

Once these deep-seated chronic ulcers have formed, it is difficult to effect normal skin healing and architecture. The underlying problem of paralysis with lack of sensation still exists and cannot be corrected; therefore, pressure necrosis is always a distinct possibility. Appropriate padding on the wheelchair and education concerning avoidance of hard surfaces while seated will be the mainstay of therapy. Evidence of infection may warrant antibiotic therapy.

Progressive Therapeutic Option

1. Education concerning appropriate padding to protect the ischial tuberosities and the pubic rami when seated.

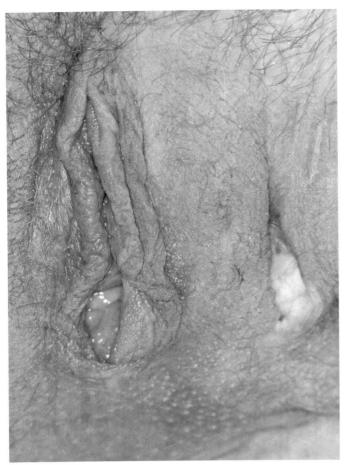

Figure 8.11. Decubitus ulcer overlying the left ischial tuberosity in a paraplegic patient. An identical lesion was present over the right ischial tuberosity.

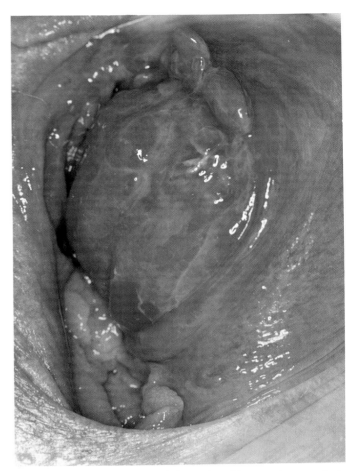

Figure 8.12. Decubitus ulcer inferior to the pubic ramus in a paraplegic woman who commonly straddles the arm rest of her wheel chair.

Herpesvirus Infection

DEFINITION

An acute, recurrent, or chronic inflammatory process caused by the herpes simplex virus (HSV).

GENERAL FEATURES

Herpes simplex is a double-stranded DNA virus belonging to the same family as varicella-zoster, cytomegalovirus, and Epstein-Barr virus. Two serotypes of HSV exist: HSV-1 and HSV-2. Although HSV-2 is more commonly associated with genital infection, HSV-1 may also be a pathogen for the vulva. Herpes simplex virus is considered a sexually transmitted disease; however, infection can be acquired by other direct contact. The herpesvirus is the most common cause of vulvar infectious ulcers in the United States. It most commonly affects adolescent and young, sexually active people.

CLINICAL PRESENTATION

There are three clinical HSV disease states: initial primary infection, initial nonprimary infection, and recurrent infection. Initial primary infections occur in patients who have never been exposed to HSV and do not possess protective antibodies. The clinical manifestations of the virus typically will occur after 3–7 days of incubation. Initial symptoms of pruritus and burning will be followed in 24–72 hours by the occurrence of a vesicular eruption on the vulva. The vesicles may continue to present over a number of days. Rupture of these vesicles will result in diffuse ulcerations, which may coalesce. These ulcerations are exquisitely painful. Systemic symptoms consist of fever, headache, and malaise. Usually there will be viral infection of the urethra and bladder and dysuria will be a common symptom in primary infections. This may progress to urinary retention. Primary lesions will usually persist for 2–6 weeks, followed by healing without scar formation. Immunocompromised patients, including patients with AIDS, may develop a disseminated infection that frequently ends in death. Multiple extragenital herpetic lesions and significant systemic symptoms should alert the clinician to this possibility. Chronic herpes infection also may occur in these patients usually presenting as a chronic, nonhealing ulcer or ulcers. Culture of such ulcers for herpesvirus is usually diagnostic.

Patients with nonprimary, first-episode herpes and patients with recurrent disease will have significantly less discomfort and less evidence of systemic disease than patients with initial primary disease. Patients with nonprimary, first-episode infections will have been infected subclinically at some point in the past and have circulating antibodies to HSV. These circulating antibodies will ameliorate the disease process. The vulvar manifestations may be so minor as to be unobserved in both nonprimary initial infections and recurrent infections. Painful ulcers usually will be present, but generally will not be as widespread as with primary episodes. The ulcers will not persist beyond 1–2 weeks in an immune competent person.

Occasionally, secondary to autoinoculation, the disease may be discovered in additional body sites other than the vulva. Of particular note is involvement of the fingers, buttocks and oral-labial mucosa. The latter may be secondary to oral-genital sex with an infected partner.

The diagnosis is suspected in all patients with vulvar ulcerations. Initial primary infections with significant systemic symptoms are classic in appearance. Nonprimary initial infections and recurrent infections may be so minor as to elude the clinician's observant eye. Confirmation of diagnosis is imperative for initiation of therapy and for appropriate preventative counseling.

MICROSCOPIC FEATURES

Acute herpesvirus infection within the epithelium is characterized by epithelial nuclear changes that are seen first as homogenization of the nuclear chromatin of the epithelial keratinocyte, giving a "ground-glass" appearance. The keratinocytes become multinucleated and, as the virus replicates within the nucleus, eosinophilic intranuclear inclusions are evident. With cell death there is karyorrhexis and cell lysis with release of the assembled viral particles into the vesicle and onto the epithelial surface when ulceration occurs. The intraepithelial vesicle contains predominately acellular fluid and is lined by epithelial cells that show viral cytopathologic changes. These changes are most evident along the epithelial edge of the vesicle. The ulcerated vesicle has an eroded epithelium with an acute and chronic inflammatory infiltrate that involves the dermis or submucosa beneath the ulcer. At this stage the typical viral cytopathologic findings may not be evident, although immunoperoxidase techniques for herpesvirus antigen may demonstrate the presence of virus within the intact epithelial cells as well as within endothelial cells. The histopathologic features cannot distinguish a primary from a secondary herpesvirus infection, nor can Herpes type 1 or 2 infections be distinguished by morphologic appearance alone.

ADJUNCTIVE STUDIES

Although Tzanck smears and Pap smears may be used for the initial clinical evaluation, the standard of diagnosis is culture of the herpesvirus. In addition to culture, monoclonal antibodies to herpesvirus can be employed in immunofluorescent or immunoperoxidase techniques to identify the virus within tissue. Polymerase-chain reaction can also be used to identify herpesvirus.

Viral culture for herpesvirus should be obtained on all patients with vulvar ulcerations. The greatest recovery rate will be noted in those lesions that are in their vesicular stages. Early ulcerative lesions will also return high positive recovery rates but ulcers of longer duration may frequently be noted to be negative (82% recovery rate for ulcerative primary lesions and 43% recovery rate for ulcerative recurrent lesions). It is therefore imperative to culture the lesion early in the course of the disease. Although serologic studies for antibody titer may be obtained, this may be helpful only in differentiating those patients who have initial primary lesions from those who have initial nonprimary lesions. This is not usually clinically germane and is therefore not cost-effective. The presumptive diagnosis of HSV infection is usually made upon clinical evaluation and definitive diagnosis awaits culture result. For the patient who presents after several days or weeks of discomfort, culture results may be falsely negative.

DIFFERENTIAL DIAGNOSIS

It is important to consider the differential diagnosis of vulvar ulcerations and obtain appropriate evaluation in addition to herpes cultures. One must consider the possibility of a primary syphilitic infection. Although chancres are classically nontender, superimposed infection may result in tenderness. Dark-field or immunofluorescent examination and serologic studies for syphilis should be obtained. HIV may be a cause of primary vulvar ulceration and should be considered in the differential diagnosis. Likewise, the immunocompromised patient with a herpetic infection may be at increased risk for disseminated herpesvirus infection or secondary infection and this information should be available to the treating physician. Behçet's disease may present with vulvar ulcerations, oral ulcerations, and visual disturbances. There are no serologic assays for Behçet's disease and clinical diag-

nosis is based upon the international classification system for Behçet's disease. Pemphigus and pemphigoid may present with vulvar ulcerations and the diagnosis will be based upon histologic and immunohistologic studies. Chancroid is an uncommon finding in the United States, but may also present with vulvar ulcerations that are tender.

CLINICAL BEHAVIOR AND TREATMENT

Acute herpesvirus infection involving the genital tract will typically heal, without scar formation, within 6 weeks. Recurrent (nonprimary) episodes of infection are common and may occur for years following the primary infection. The severity and duration of the recurrent episodes typically decrease over time until the patient becomes asymptomatic.

Initial treatment of the patient with herpes vulvar disease is based upon control of the symptoms. Analgesics and antipruritics may be necessary to control systemic manifestations of primary infections. Urinary retention will often require placement of a suprapubic catheter. Intraurethral catheters will be uncomfortable due to the urethral irritation caused by the primary infection. If a transurethral catheter is used for bladder drainage, appropriate topical anesthetic gel should be placed on the catheter and urethra prior to insertion. Cool soaks will augment the analgesic effect of orally administered analgesics. Salt-water sitz baths may be beneficial. Therapy with acyclovir is indicated in primary infections. The dose is 200 mg five times a day for approximately 7–10 days. Alternatively the drug may be administered as 400 mg three times a day as a more convenient dosing form. Patients with significant systemic symptoms or findings who are incapable of taking oral acyclovir or who are suspected of having disseminated disease should be admitted to receive intravenous acyclovir at 5 mg/kg every 8 hours for 5–7 days. For immunocompromised patients higher dosages or oral therapy are recommended for moderate disease (400 mg 5 times a day) and hospitalization should be strongly considered with suspicion of disease dissemination.

Treatment for recurrent genital herpes is 200 mg of acyclovir orally five times a day for 5 days, provided the infection is noted early in the disease state. If therapy is initiated early for recurrent genital herpes then viral shedding may be reduced and the duration of the episode may be reduced as well.

For the patient with significant recurrent disease, prophylactic use of acyclovir may be considered. This may be administered as 400 mg twice daily. The decision to initiate acyclovir prophylaxis should be based upon a reasonable assessment of the patient's number of recurrences. It would be less than cost-effective to initiate therapy for one episode of recurrence per year. It is also imperative that patients use safe and efficient contraception while taking prophylactic acyclovir. Acyclovir may be continued for 12 months, at which time reassessment must be considered. Long-term side effects of acyclovir remain to be defined. The potential for side effects versus benefits should be weighed. The possibility of acyclovir resistance must also be considered. With chronic use of acyclovir, especially in immunocompromised patients, emergence of resistant strains of herpesvirus may have significant implications for the patient.

Patients should be advised that asymptomatic viral shedding may occur at any time in the absence of clinically obvious herpes lesions. Patients should abstain from any form of direct contact when obvious lesions are present and should use barrier contraception with contraceptive foams or gels possessing antiherpetic activity. Patients will often require extensive counseling concerning the future ramifications of what will be a lifelong infection with the herpesvirus. It should be clear to the patient that the herpesvirus will reside in a dormant state in the dorsal root ganglia of S-2, S-3, and S-4 and may recur at any time because of unknown factors. Stress should be placed upon the potential risk for a future pregnancy delivered through a birth canal with an obvious herpetic lesion. Neonatal infection with herpes has a high mortality rate.

Progressive Therapeutic Options

1. Initial primary infection: acyclovir 200 mg orally five times a day for 7–10 days or 400 mg orally three times a day for convenience for 7–10 days. Oral analgesics and antipruritics for systemic symptoms. Suprapubic or urethral catheterization for urinary retention.

2. For recurrent herpes: acyclovir 200 mg orally five times a day for 5 days or 400 mg orally three times daily for 5 days (for convenience). Prophylaxis for recurrent herpes of significant impact: acyclovir 400 mg two times a day for 1 year and reassess and counsel patient appropriately. Appropriate effective contraception should be mandatory when taking prophylactic acyclovir.

3. For the immunocompromised patient (AIDS): With moderate primary disease consider increasing the acyclovir dose to 400 mg five times a day and determine length of therapy by response.

4. For the HIV-positive patient with evidence of disseminated mucocutaneous herpes genitalis: hospitalize for intravenous acyclovir.

5. For patients with disseminated primary herpes, administer acyclovir intravenously at 5 mg/kg every 8 hours for 5–7 days or longer depending upon clinical response.

NOTATION: Obtain an HIV assay after appropriate counseling on all patients with vulvar ulcerations.

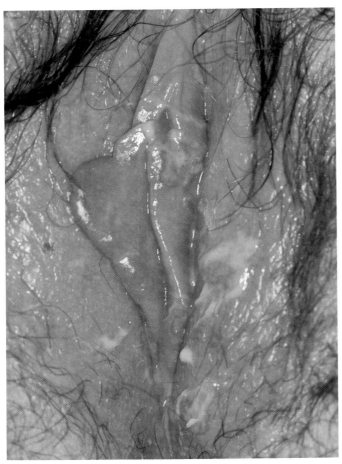

Figure 8.13. Multiple tender ulcers of uncertain duration, culture positive for HSV type 2. Acyclovir therapy was instituted for primary herpes. Patient has monthly recurrences for 5–7 days.

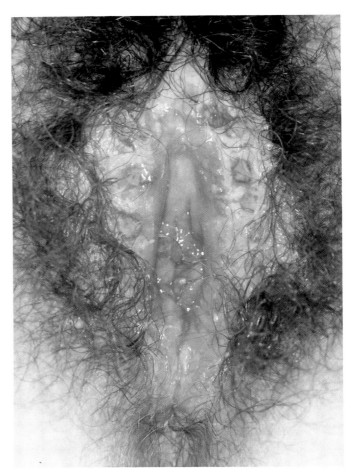

Figure 8.14. Multiple tender ulcers of approximately 3 days' duration associated with fever and dysuria. The culture was positive for HSV type 1. Acyclovir therapy was instituted for primary herpes. No recurrence has been noted for 8 months.

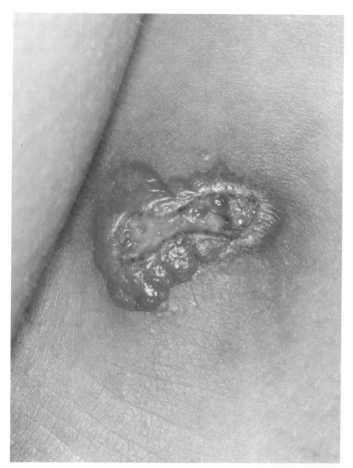

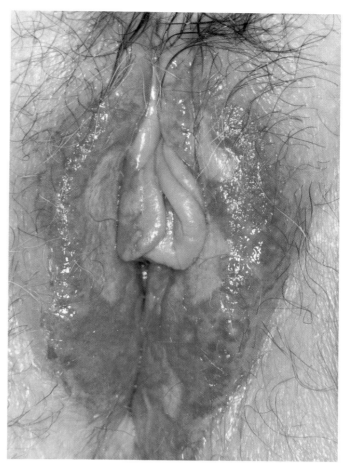

Figure 8.15. A lesion on the buttock of an HIV-positive patient. The ulcer has been present for 7 months and is, upon evaluation, culture-positive for HSV. Prompt resolution of the ulcer occurred with initiation of acyclovir therapy.

Figure 8.16. Herpes present for 2.5 months in a patient with pancyto-penia and an unknown HIV status.

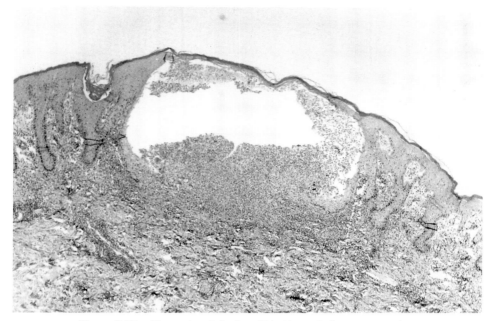

Figure 8.17. Herpesvirus infection. This biopsy is from a regressing vesicle. Necrosis with acute inflammation is evident in the epithelium. The viral changes are found at the edge of the intraepithelial abscess.

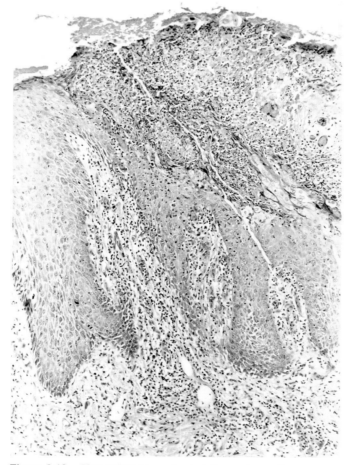

Figure 8.18. Herpesvirus ulcer. Acute inflammatory cells are present in the adjacent tissues.

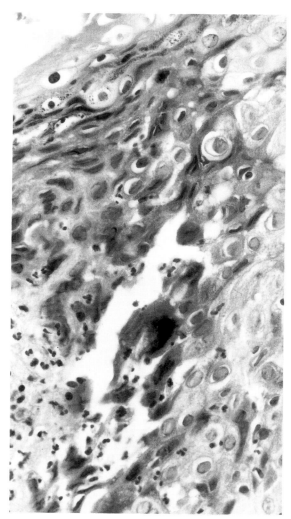

Figure 8.19. Herpesvirus infection. A higher magnification of the herpes ulcer demonstrates the viral epithelial changes. The nuclear chromatin of some of the involved keratinocytes is clear, and others have typical intranuclear inclusions.

Hidradenitis Suppurativa

DEFINITION

Hidradenitis suppurativa is a chronic, often debilitating, disease initiated by obstruction and subsequent inflammation of apocrine glands with resultant sinus tract and abscess formation.

GENERAL FEATURES

The etiology of hidradenitis suppurativa is unknown but there appears to be a familial tendency, suggesting a genetic predisposition. Hypersensitivity to androgens has been suggested as a possible etiology. The disease has not been noted before the onset of puberty, supporting a relationship to androgen levels. Bacteria abound in the affected tissues and the most commonly isolated organisms are staphylococci, streptococci, and anaerobes. These are not necessarily initiators of the process but are more probably secondary invaders.

CLINICAL PRESENTATIONS

Patients may present at any age after the onset of puberty with a complaint of discomfort in apocrine gland-bearing skin. Most commonly affected areas are the axillae, vulva, and perineum. The patient with vulvar hidradenitis suppurativa may have extragenital involvement in one or more of these areas. Early disease commonly presents as a localized abscess. With progression of the disease, there is extensive sinus tract formation with multiple abscesses and significant scarring with loss of normal architecture. Intercourse may be extremely uncomfortable and even impossible secondary to the inflammatory reaction in the vulvar skin.

MICROSCOPIC FINDINGS

On microscopic examination the early stages of hidradenitis suppurativa are characterized by a perifolliculitis with an associated acute and chronic dermal inflammatory infiltrate. With more advanced disease the predominant features are of a chronic inflammatory process within in the subcutaneous tissues that involves and is associated with destruction of the adjacent skin appendages. Ulcerated epidermis is found overlying subcutaneous abscesses. The abscesses are typically multiple and communicate with subcutaneous sinuses. Fibrosis and scarring with loss of skin appendages is usually evident.

HISTOCHEMICAL AND IMMUNOHISTOCHEMICAL FINDINGS

Special stains for organisms, including acid fast stain, silver stains for spirochetes, fungi, and bacteria, as well as bacterial stains typically do not demonstrate organisms within the inflamed tissues.

DIFFERENTIAL DIAGNOSIS

Advanced vulvar hidradenitis suppurativa may be confused with vulvar Crohn's disease. A point of clinical differentiation is that vulvar Crohn's disease is primarily an ulcerative process. Ulcers noted with vulvar Crohn's disease may be extensive and deeply seated and frequently follow a linear distribution lateral to the labia majora. Vulvar Crohn's disease has been observed concomitantly in patients with hidradenitis suppurativa. It is important to obtain a complete history concerning bowel symptoms that might suggest inflammatory bowel disease and would necessitate further evaluation endoscopically to rule out Crohn's disease. Fox-Fordyce disease may resemble hidradenitis suppurativa, or may occur with it; however, there are intraepithelial vesicles and associated dilated apocrine ducts with dermal chronic inflammation associated with mucin positive secretion within the ducts and adjacent tissues. Fox-Fordyce disease is associated with plugging of the intraepithelial portion of the sweat duct resulting in a dilated duct within the epidermis with formation of intraepithelial vesicles. The dissection of the sweat within the dermis may be evident. Deep subcutaneous sinuses are typically not found.

Lymphogranuloma venereum may result in anogenital findings that may be indistinguishable from hidradenitis suppurativa. The classic groove sign described in patients with lymphogranuloma venereum also may be seen in patients with hidradenitis suppurativa. The inguinal nodes and inflamed skin may project above the inguinal ligament in both conditions, resulting in this nonspecific finding. A serologic assay for chlamydia should be obtained. It is interesting that patients with hidradenitis suppurativa may have an elevated chlamydia serotiter. Uncertainty exists concerning whether this reflects an etiologic relationship. It may be that the association is purely coincidental because chlamydia is one of the most prevalent sexually transmitted diseases in modern society.

Vulvar biopsy occasionally may be warranted to arrive at a correct diagnosis. Typically this will not be necessary, especially in the patient with axillary manifestations of hidradenitis suppurativa in addition to the vulvar disease.

CLINICAL BEHAVIOR AND TREATMENT

The patient who presents with minor vulvar manifestations of hidradenitis suppurativa may be managed with relatively simple pharmacologic intervention. The first order of systemic therapy is initiation of oral contraceptive use. It is widely accepted that oral contraceptives increase sex hormone binding globulins and therefore decrease the amount of free testosterone available to affect androgen sensitive skin. The newer oral contraceptives containing desogestrel and ethinyl estradiol may be more advantageous in managing this androgen-sensitive condition, although no prospective studies exist.

Oral or topical antibiotics directed against the most commonly isolated organisms may be efficacious in managing minor hidradenitis suppurativa. If patients have been placed on oral contraceptives they should be forewarned that the contraceptive effectiveness of the hormone preparation may be diminished by the concomitant use of antibiotics. Tetracyclines in the range of 2 grams per day may be used for long-term management of hidradenitis suppurativa. Alternatively, topical clindamycin applied daily may diminish the inflammatory response.

With advancing persistent active disease under the above management, consideration should be given to more aggressive therapy. Isotretinoin (Accutane) is on occasion efficacious in managing more advanced hidradenitis suppurativa. The dosage used is 1 mg/kg/day. Patients should be counseled extensively concerning the teratogenic effects of isotretinoin and oral contraceptive therapy should be initiated unless contraindicated. Patients should be monitored regularly with liver function tests, cholesterol and triglyceride levels and complete blood cell counts.

Success has been reported with oral use of dexamethasone to suppress the adrenal contribution to androgen levels. Likewise gonadotropin-releasing hormone agonist therapy (leuprolide) has demonstrated an ameliorative affect on hidradenitis suppurativa. With discontinuation of these medications the disease state will usually return to its pretherapy level. In addition, agents such as gonadotropin-releasing hormone agonists will result in significant financial costs.

Small abscesses may be drained and the patient may be counseled concerning vulvar hygiene with emphasis on maintaining the skin in as dry a state as possible. For advanced hidradenitis suppurativa the most efficacious therapy is wide surgical excision. Attempts to manage advanced disease pharmacologically are almost invariably disappointing. Extensive disease may be removed as a staged procedure or as a single wide local excision. All inflamed tissue in the apocrine gland-bearing region should be removed to decrease the probability of recurrence. This may require deep dissection to the fascia. Healing has been acceptable with secondary intention, although split-thickness skin grafts may be used after the surgical bed is free of devitalized or infected tissue. Postoperative management of patients who have undergone wide local excision may require prolonged hospitalization with frequent whirlpool baths and frequent dressing changes. Diverting colostomy is rarely necessary. The patient should be forewarned of the prolonged recovery period and the need for meticulous hygiene until complete healing is accomplished. Recurrences of disease outside of the excised area may be managed with local excision.

An alternative to wide local excision is use of the CO_2 laser to destroy abscessed skin and unroof and vaporize sinus tracts. Patients should be counseled that areas of postinflammatory depigmentation and scarring may be noted after healing is completed. Healing is primarily by secondary intent.

The role of immunosuppressant therapy in the management of hidradenitis suppurativa remains relatively uncertain and uninvestigated. Until the role of immunosuppression is further defined in this disease condition, its use should be considered investigational.

Progressive Therapeutic Options

1. Incision and drainage of localized abscesses with emphasis on vulvar hygiene and control of perspiration.
2. Initiation of oral contraceptive therapy (estrogen-progestin combination).
3. Initiation of oral antibiotic therapy (most commonly tetracyclines).
4. Isotretinoin (Accutane) 1 mg/kg/day (two divided doses) with appropriate counseling concerning teratogenicity and **initiation of contra-**

ceptive therapy most commonly with oral contraceptives. Monthly evaluations of blood parameters (complete blood cell counts, liver function tests, cholesterol, triglycerides).

5. Surgical intervention with wide local excision and healing by secondary intent. CO_2 laser vaporization may be considered an alternative or ancillary approach for localized disease.

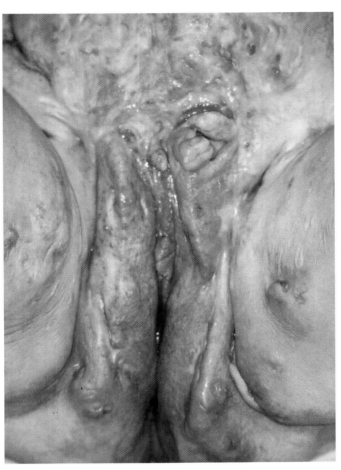

Figure 8.20. Multiple sinus tracts and ulcers in a patient with hidradenitis diagnosed initially in axillae 9 years previously.

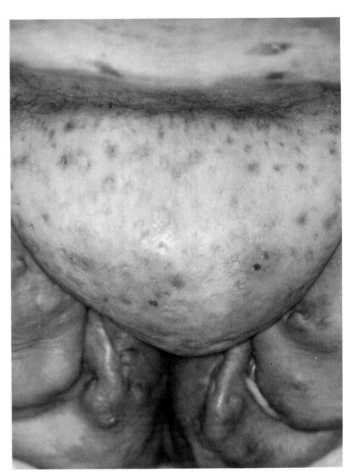

Figure 8.21. Edematous mons involved with hidradenitis.

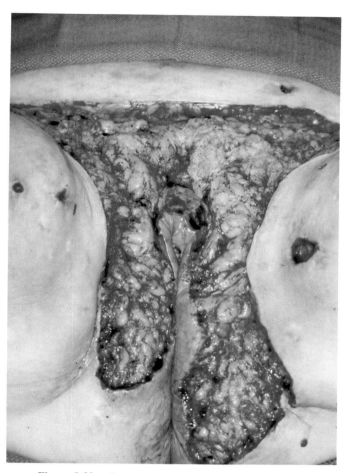

Figure 8.22. Surgical excision of vulva, including mons.

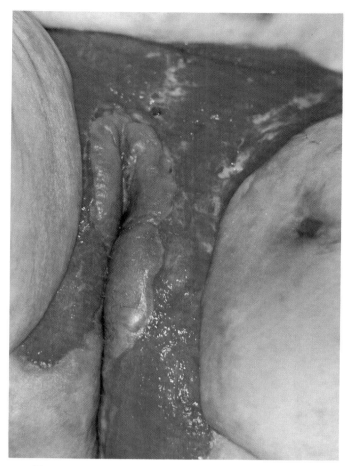

Figure 8.23. Granulation tissue 4 weeks after vulvectomy.

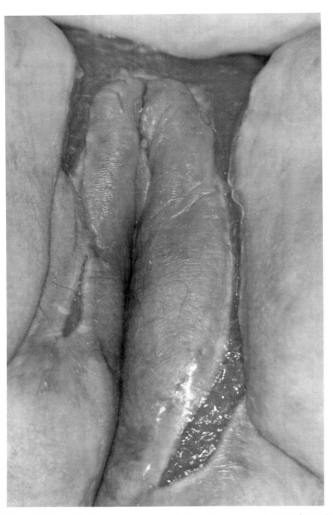

Figure 8.24. Healing by secondary intent almost complete at 8 weeks after vulvectomy.

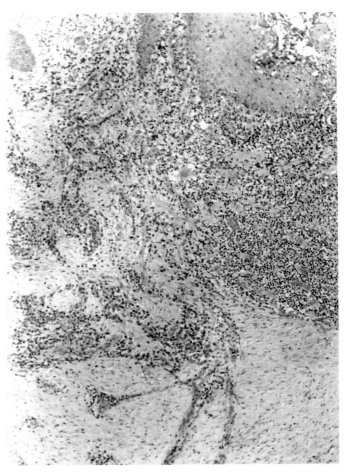

Figure 8.25. Hidradenitis suppurativa. There is severe superficial and deep inflammation with perifolliculitis. The adjacent skin appendages are involved in the inflammatory process and a sinus tract is present.

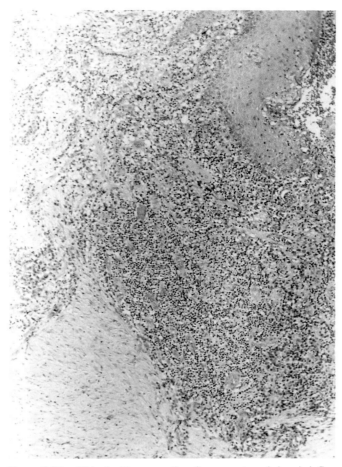

Figure 8.26. Hidradenitis suppurativa. Severe acute and chronic inflammation is present about the apocrine glands of the deep dermis.

Lymphogranuloma Venereum

DEFINITION

Lymphogranuloma venereum (LGV) is a sexually transmitted disease caused by the L-1, L-2, and L-3 serotypes of *Chlamydia trachomatis*.

GENERAL FEATURES

LGV is most commonly seen in tropical and subtropical regions and is an uncommon disease in the United States.

CLINICAL PRESENTATION

LGV has three relatively distinct stages of clinical presentation. In the first stage a genital vesicle or papule is observed that may progress to a painless ulcer approximately 3–10 days after inoculation. Unless the patient palpates this lesion, it will usually go unnoticed. The lesion is usually noted on the posterior aspect of the vulva or vestibule but may be found in the vagina or cervix. Patients engaging in anal intercourse may present with proctitis with associated tenesmus and bloody discharge or diarrhea. The primary vulvar ulceration or vesicle may heal rapidly and over the ensuing months the secondary stage will evolve. During this stage the lymphatic vessels and nodes become inflamed. Depending upon the initial location of the genital lesion, specific regional nodes will be involved. Lymph nodes in the inguinal region are less frequently involved in women than in men. Involvement may be unilateral or bilateral. As the lymph nodes enlarge the inguinal ligament will maintain its original anatomic position, resulting in a groove-like appearance, the so-called "groove sign." The groove sign is not specific for lymphogranuloma venereum and may be observed in other diseases causing regional adenopathy, such as hidradenitis suppurativa. Lymph nodes may abscess, rupture, and drain. This process will result in chronic draining sinus tracts. Drainage to regional nodes posteriorly may result in abscessed nodes that may not be clinically apparent. The patient may present with severe pain in the lower abdomen and pelvis. Systemic symptoms, such as fever, may be present.

With continued involvement of the lymph nodes and lymph channels, fibrosis and scarring will result in genital edema. This third stage of LGV is associated with elephantiasis of the vulva, to which the term "esthiomene" is applied. Draining sinus tracts and rectal strictures associated with this anogenital syndrome will be debilitating and, depending upon the severity of the anal strictures, may be life threatening.

Patients are rarely seen in the initial stage of the disease. The low prevalence of this disease in the United States would rarely lead to its inclusion in the differential diagnosis of the primary lesion. A high index of suspicion will be the clinician's greatest aid in diagnosis. Most commonly the diagnosis is made by serologic assay. Although complement fixation assays are nonspecific and reflect chlamydial infection from a number of different serotypes, a titer greater than 1:64 is considered highly suggestive of LGV in a patient with the appropriate clinical presentation. A more specific microimmunofluorescent antibody assay for the specific serotypes associated with LGV is available in reference laboratories, but is not generally available in most hospital settings. Rarely, material may be aspirated from abscessed lymph nodes, through intact normal skin, and submitted for culture on McCoy cells. Open biopsy of these nodes should be avoided because the biopsy or excision site will result in a chronic draining sinus. It must be remembered that the diagnosis should be suspected in patients with perirectal abscess formation and rectal/anal strictures. Although the patient with a significant stricture may require a diverting colostomy and appropriate biopsies to rule out carcinoma, preoperative serologic testing positive for LGV would have major implications for future intervention and therapy.

MICROSCOPIC FINDINGS

LGV has no morphologically distinctive features. The primary ulcer of LGV is rarely recognized, but if biopsied, is not diagnostic unless cultures are performed. LGV must be considered when a superficial and deep chronic inflammatory infiltrate, consisting predominately of lymphocytes, plasma cells, and some giant cells, is identified. Advanced lesions may be associated with sinus tract formation and severe dermal fibrosis. Organisms are not identifiable in the lesion by conventional light microscopy. Clinical and pathologic findings suggesting LGV should be followed up with cultures for LGV and complement fixation tests.

Lymph nodes enlarged secondary to LGV usually are not biopsied; however, fine-needle aspiration for culture and cytologic evaluation can be diagnostic. Incisional drainage or excision of such nodes is generally contraindicated in that incision can lead to a chronically draining groin ulcer.

CLINICAL BEHAVIOR AND TREATMENT

The initial stages of LGV are treated with oral tetracycline in a dose of 500 mg 4 times a day for approximately 3 weeks. Based upon response, therapy may be necessary for longer periods of time. Alternative regimens would include doxycycline 100 mg twice a day for a similar length of time. The patient who is allergic to tetracyclines or who is pregnant may take 500 mg of erythromycin 4 times a day. An alternative regimen is sulfadiazine 1 g 4 times a day for 14–21 days after an initial 2-g loading dose. Again, duration of therapy will be dictated by response to pharmacologic intervention.

Bubos should not be incised and drained. This surgical procedure will result in sinus tract formation. Drainage, when necessary, should be via needle aspiration through normal skin and should be accomplished to prevent rupture of large, tense bubos. Patients with strictures of the rectum may require diverting bowel procedures to permit appropriate evacuation of bowel contents.

Progressive Therapeutic Options

1. Doxycycline 100 mg orally twice daily for 21 days or tetracycline 500 mg orally four times daily for 21 days or erythromycin 500 mg orally four times daily for 21 days or sulfadiazine 1 g orally four times daily (after a 2-g loading dose) for 21 days.

NOTATION: Patients who are pregnant should not be exposed to tetracyclines.

2. Needle aspiration of tense bubos through normal skin, to prevent rupture and subsequent sinus formation, for cytologic diagnosis and culture.
3. Surgical management of chronic debilitating third-stage anogenital syndrome after initiating a thorough course of antibiotic therapy.
4. Diverting bowel procedure for the patient with significant anogenital syndrome and severe rectal stricture formation resulting in obstipation. Appropriate antibiotic coverage for lymphogranuloma venereum and secondary microbial agents is required.

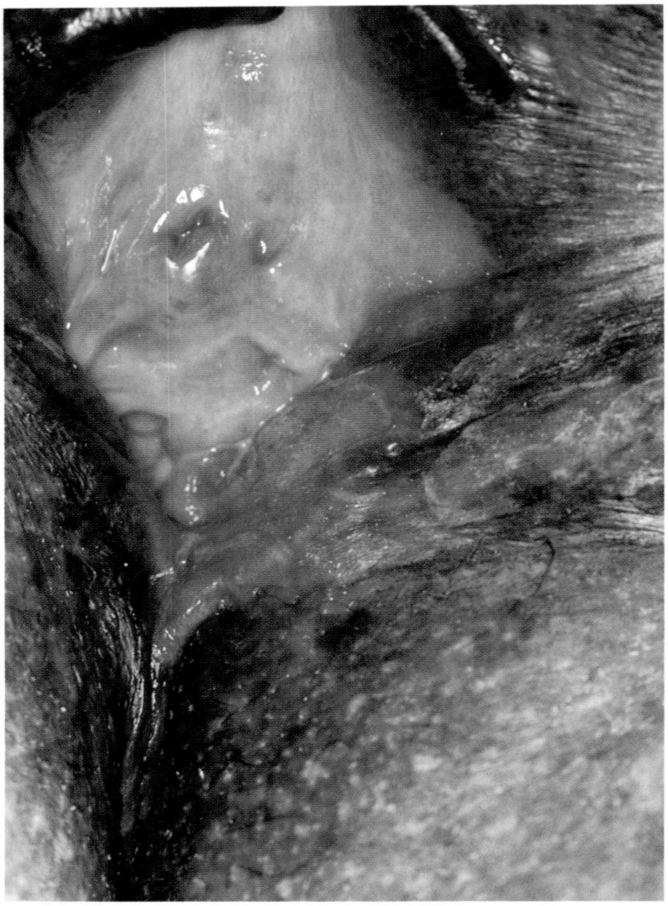

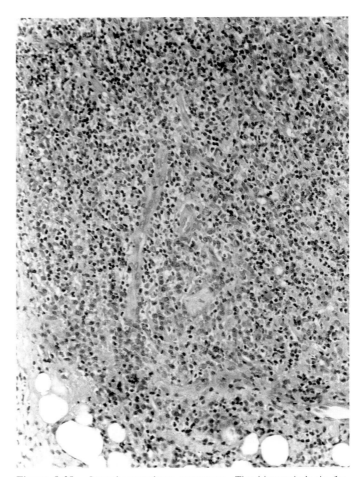

Figure 8.27. Painful ulcer present for several months. Biopsy demonstrated intense inflammation. Immunofluorescent studies were nonspecific. *Chlamydia* serology was positive (1:128). The ulcer resolved after 3 weeks of doxycycline.

Figure 8.28. Lymphogranuloma venereum. The histopathologic features of LGV consist of a deep and superficial chronic inflammatory infiltrate that is composed predominantly of lymphocytes and plasma cells with some giant cells. The histologic features are not diagnostic alone and culture as well as specific immunohistologic studies are needed for definitive diagnosis.

Pemphigoid

DEFINITION

Pemphigoid is a subepidermal autoimmune blistering disease most commonly seen in elderly or middle-aged patients.

CLINICAL PRESENTATION

Vulvar presentation of pemphigoid is uncommon. When vulvar and vaginal lesions are noted, the suspicion should be that one is dealing with cicatricial pemphigoid rather than bullous pemphigoid. Cicatricial pemphigoid has a greater tendency to involve mucous membranes, whereas bullous pemphigoid more commonly involves skin and rarely involves mucous membranes. The vulva and vagina may be the only anatomic regions involved initially with pemphigoid. Disease progression may eventuate in lesions in the mouth, skin, and eyes. The most common presentation of pemphigoid in the vulvovaginal region is the occurrence of blisters on the vulva. These blisters may have the appearance of pustules and indeed the suspicion may be that one is dealing with folliculitis. Vaginal examination may demonstrate desquamating vaginal epithelium. Pressure on the cervix or vaginal walls may result in desquamation of epithelium. Fragile epithelium that readily denudes is denoted as a positive Nikolsky's sign. Although Nikolsky's sign is most commonly seen with pemphigus, in the vagina it may be observed with pemphigoid as well. Oral lesions are a further manifestation of the desquamative process. Transient ulcerations of the gingival and buccal mucosa may be observed. Blistering skin lesions in cicatricial pemphigoid usually will heal with scarring. Eye involvement may manifest itself as unilateral or bilateral conjunctivitis. With progression of disease, severe scarring may eventuate in blindness. Laryngeal and esophageal lesions resulting in stenosis also may occur.

The diagnosis of vulvovaginal pemphigoid is based upon strong clinical suspicion of the disease. Biopsy of the vulvar lesion will assist in defining whether one is dealing with an intraepidermal or a subepidermal blistering disease, thus assisting in differentiation between pemphigus and pemphigoid. In addition to routine histologic studies, direct immunofluorescent studies should be obtained. The final diagnosis is based upon (*a*) scarring blisters, (*b*) subepithelial blistering on histologic examinations, and (*c*) direct immunofluorescent studies demonstrating IgG and complement deposited along the basement membrane. Biopsies should be obtained from perilesional epithelium because lesional epithelium will often peel, making the direct immunofluorescent studies difficult to read. Not all patients will be positive on direct immunofluorescence, and clinical suspicion should remain high for cicatricial pemphigoid even in the absence of a positive direct immunofluorescent study, provided the other histologic and clinical manifestations are present. Indirect immunofluorescent studies typically will be negative. It is advisable to obtain such studies if the possibility of pemphigus is being entertained. Circulating autoantibodies frequently are positive in patients who have pemphigus.

MICROSCOPIC FINDINGS

The blisters, or larger bullae, of bullous pemphigoid are subepidermal and there is a dermal inflammatory infiltrate that consists of acute and chronic inflammatory cells. Immunofluorescent studies, by the direct method, demonstrate IgG deposited in a linear manner within the basement membrane. IgA and IgM immunoglobulin as well as complement C_3 and C_5 also may be found, but this is not a consistent finding. A knowledge of clinical history and physical findings is essential to distinguish bullous from cicatricial pemphigoid.

CLINICAL BEHAVIOR AND TREATMENT

Cicatricial pemphigoid typically is associated with small blisters and erosions that often lead to vulvar, vaginal, and perineal scarring and shrinkage, unlike bullous pemphigoid. Cicatricial pemphigoid may be drug related. Concurrent, known, or subsequent ocular involvement also may occur.

Therapy for pemphigoid localized to the vulvovaginal region and is not extensive may be initiated with topical steroid preparations. Short courses of superpotent steroids such as halobetasol (Ultravate) or clobetasol (Temovate) may alleviate discomfort noted on the vulva. More frequently, oral prednisone will be required. Therapy will usually start at 60 mg of prednisone per day with subsequent tapering. With resolution of the disease process, steroids may be discontinued; however, it will be necessary to maintain the patient on chronic, low-dose steroids if complete resolution is not observed. To decrease steroid requirements, Dapsone may be added at 50 mg/day and the dose may be increased by 50-mg increments over successive weeks (maximum 200–250 mg/day). Before initiating Dapsone a glucose-6-phosphate dehydrogenase (G-6-PD) screen should be obtained. Patients who have a G-6-PD deficiency may hemolyze red blood cells while taking Dapsone, and it would be strongly advised to avoid Dapsone. Patients who are taking Dapsone should be followed regularly with complete blood cell counts. An occasional patient will become anemic even with a negative G-6-PD screen. Although niacinamide and tetracycline have been used to treat bullous pemphigoid, success has not been reported in treating cicatricial pemphigoid with this regimen.

In patients who do not respond to oral prednisone or Dapsone, immunosuppressant therapy may be necessary. If ocular involvement is noted, cyclophosphamide is the most efficacious immunosuppressant. The dose required is 1–2 mg/kg/day for 18–24 months. Most patients will have clinical remission on this regimen; however, it will be necessary to follow blood cell counts throughout the course of therapy. An alternate form of therapy, with fewer side effects, and fewer long-term concerns is use of azathioprine (Imuran). This agent may be used for vulvovaginal cicatricial pemphigoid not involving the eye or other organ systems and unresponsive to prednisone and/or Dapsone. Although higher dosages in the range of 3–5 mg/kg/day are used for transplant patients, it would be prudent to begin at a lower dose, in the range of 1 mg/kg/day, to determine response and level of toxicity. After 6–8 weeks the dose may be increased if needed. It may take several weeks to see an obvious response. Patients should be followed with complete blood cell counts, liver function tests, and serum amylase and lipase levels. With evidence of unacceptable toxicity the medication should be discontinued. An additional immunosuppressant to be considered is cyclosporine. Concern exists about the long-term effect of cyclosporine on renal function, and minimal experience exists with the use of this agent in treating cicatricial pemphigoid.

Progressive Therapeutic Options

1. Topical medium-strength steroids (betamethasone 0.1%) or short courses of topical superpotent steroids (halobetasol or clobetasol 0.05%).
2. Dapsone 50 mg/day after obtaining a negative G-6-PD screen. Dose may be increased by 50-mg increments to maximum of 200–250 mg/day. Complete blood cell count should be followed.
3. Trial of tetracycline 1–2 g/day with niacinamide 1–2 g/day if uncertainty exists concerning diagnosis (bullous pemphigoid vs cicatricial pemphigoid). Bullous pemphigoid is more likely to respond.
4. Systemic steroids at 60 mg/day orally with tapering after the disease activity decreases.
5. Azathioprine (Imuran) should be added at 1–2 mg/kg/day if disease activity is marked. Prednisone may be tapered while the azathioprine dose is held constant. Follow complete blood cell counts, liver function tests, amylase and lipase.
6. Consider cyclophosphamide (1–2 mg/kg) in patients with ocular involvement.

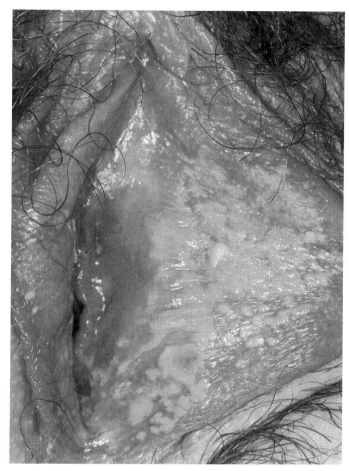

Figure 8.29. Plaquelike, painful eruption on labia minora consistent with pemphigoid on biopsy.

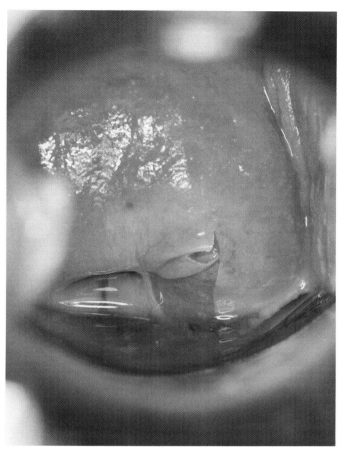

Figure 8.30. Nikolsky's sign observed on the cervix of patient with pemphigoid (Fig. 8.29). Epithelium denudes when touched due to sub-epithelial fluid.

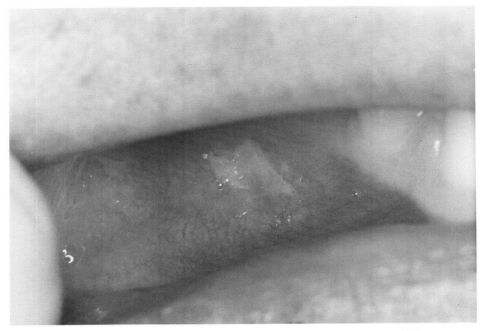

Figure 8.31.   Painful oral ulceration in patient with pemphigoid (Fig. 8.29).

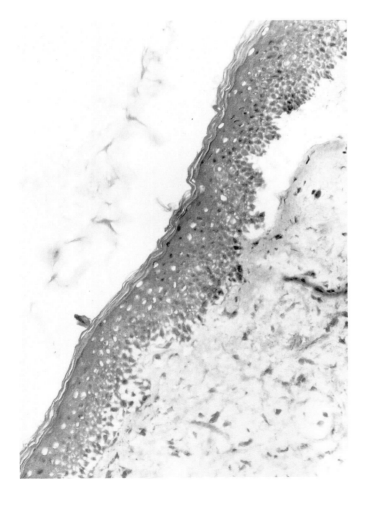

Figure 8.32.   Pemphigoid. The vesicle is subepithelial and the entire epithelium is detached from the underlying dermis. There is an acute and chronic inflammatory infiltrate within the superficial dermis.

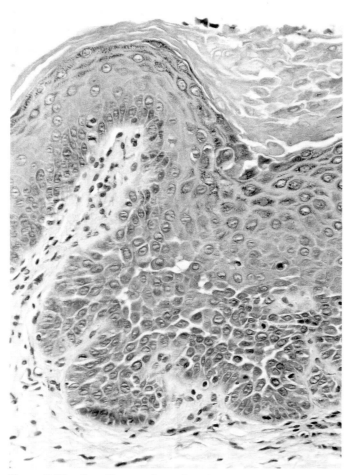

Figure 8.33. Pemphigus vegitans. Prominent acantholysis is present with suprabasal vesicle formation. Within the dermis eosinophils are typically present.

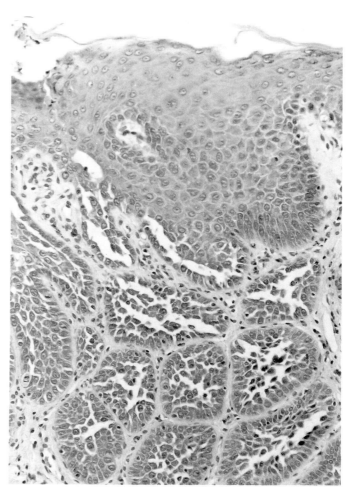

Figure 8.34. Pemphigus vulgaris. The vesicles of pemphigus vulgaris are suprabasal, with a characteristic ''picket fence'' arrangement of the residual basal cells attached to the basement membrane. In this field, adjacent to a vesicle, acantholysis with loss of intracellular bridges is evident.

Squamous Cell Carcinoma (Superficially Invasive Squamous Cell Carcinoma)

DEFINITION

A primary, solitary squamous cell carcinoma of the vulva that is 2 cm or less in diameter with a depth of invasion of 1 mm or less is classified as superficially invasive squamous cell carcinoma.

GENERAL FEATURES

The identification of a subset of superficially invasive vulvar squamous cell carcinoma that would not be at risk for metastasis to inguinal or regional lymph nodes has progressed through a series of definitions of microinvasion that have been proposed by numerous investigators. Initial studies, following work that had been done on the cervix, used 5-mm depth of invasion as the basis of separation. Using the 5-mm depth of invasion it has subsequently been found that 15.2% of these women will have inguinal lymph node metastasis. A 3-mm depth of invasion has been suggested; however, this depth of invasion was found to be associated with inguinal lymph node metastasis in 10.2% of cases (Wilkinson, 1991). With recent studies, it is now becoming evident that to establish a depth of invasion that will not be associated with inguinal lymph node metastasis, the depth of invasion cannot exceed 1 mm (Hacker, 1993).

CLINICAL FEATURES

Clinically, vulvar squamous cell carcinomas can be ulcerated, exophytic, or appear as hyperkeratotic plaques. Superficially invasive carcinomas may present associated with VIN as granular red areas or areas with ulceration or marked hyperkeratosis adjacent to a VIN lesion. Superficially invasive carcinomas are, by definition, 2 cm or less in diameter and solitary lesions. There should be no evidence of metastasis to regional lymph nodes, or any other sites.

Table 8.1
Classification of Vulvar Intraepithelial Neoplasia

Squamous intraepithelial neoplasia
VIN 1	Mild dysplasia
VIN 2	Moderate dysplasia
VIN 3	Severe dysplasia or carcinoma in situ
VIN 3	Carcinoma in situ differentiated type

Nonsquamous intraepithelial neoplasia
  Paget's disease
  Melanoma in situ

From Wilkinson EJ, Lynch PF, Kneale B. International society for the study of vulvar disease: Report of the ISSVD Terminology Committee J Reprod Med 1986;31:973–994.

Clinical staging should be conducted as directed by the International Federation of Gynecologists and Obstetricians and the Society of Gynecologic Oncology as shown in Table 8.2.

The International Society for the Study of Vulvar Disease (ISSVD) in 1983 accepted the following definition for superficially invasive squamous cell carcinoma of the vulva, a lesion that the Society suggests be called "Stage Ia carcinoma." "Stage Ia carcinoma of the vulva" is defined as a single lesion measuring 2 cm or less in diameter and with a depth of invasion of 1 mm or less. Patients with more than one site of invasion are not included in this definition (Kneale, 1983). The preferred measurement is from the epithelial stromal junction of the most adjacent dermal papillae to the deepest point of invasion (defined as the depth of invasion) (Kurman et al., 1992; Wilkinson, 1987; Wilkinson et al., 1986). This definition includes cases that have capillary-like space involvement so long as the tumor does not invade deeper than 1 mm. The term microinvasive carcinoma is not recommended for

Table 8.2
Staging of Vulvar Carcinoma (International Federation of Obstetrics and Gynecology, 1989)

Stage 0		
	Tis	Carcinoma in situ, intraepithelial carcinoma.
Stage I		
	T1, N0, M0	Tumor confined to the vulva and/or perineum, 2 cm or less in greatest dimension, nodes are not palpable.
Stage II		
	T2, N0, M0	Tumor confined to the vulva and/or perineum, more than 2 cm in greater dimension, nodes are not palpable.
Stage III		
	T3, N0, M0	Tumor of any size with
	T3, N1, M0	1. Adjacent spread to the lower urethra and/or the vagina,
	T1, N1, M0	and/or the anus, and/or
		2. Unilateral regional lymph node metastasis.
	T2, N1, M0	
Stage IVA		
	T1, N2, M0	Tumor invades any of the following:
	T2, N2, M0	Upper urethra, bladder mucosa, rectal mucosa, pelvic bone, and/or bilateral regional node metastasis.
	T3, N2, M0	
	T4, any N, M0	
Stage IVB		
	Any T	Any distant metastasis, including pelvic lymph nodes.
	Any N, M1	

Table 8.3
Histologic Types of Squamous Vulvar Carcinoma

Squamous cell carcinoma not otherwise specified
  Well differentiated
  Moderately well differentiated
  Poorly differentiated
Basaloid carcinoma
Warty (condylomatous) carcinoma
Verrucous carcinoma
Giant cell carcinoma
Spindle cell carcinoma
Acantholytic squamous cell carcinoma (adenoid squamous
  carcinoma)
Lymphoepithelioma-like carcinoma
Basal cell carcinoma
  Metatypical basal cell carcinoma (basosquamous carcinoma)
  Adenoid basal cell carcinoma
  Sebaceous cell carcinoma
Merkel cell tumor

tumors on the vulva by either the ISSVD or the International Society of Gynecological Pathologists because the term is ambiguous.

A diagnosis of superficially invasive carcinoma of the vulva cannot be established unless the entire tumor is available for study. A single small biopsy demonstrating a very shallow tumor does not preclude the tumor being deeper beyond the involved edge of the biopsy. The specimen submitted for examination is an elliptical excision of the tumor with at least a 1-cm margin. The specimen should have the deep and lateral margins marked with india ink, or other permanent marker, and the specimen should be completely sectioned and submitted in toto for histologic examination. This will ensure that the deepest area of invasion, as well as the nature of the surgical margins, can be defined.

MICROSCOPIC FINDINGS

Superficially invasive vulvar squamous cell carcinomas may be warty, basaloid, or well-differentiated keratinizing tumors. They may grow in a compact or diffuse, fingerlike, manner. The deepest point of invasion with a tumor having a diffuse pattern of growth requires meticulous search for small islands of tumor deep to the primary tumor site.

It is recommended that the following information be included in the final pathology report.

1. The depth of invasion in millimeters.
2. The thickness of the tumor.
3. The method of measurement of the depth of invasion.
4. The presence or absence of vascular space involvement by tumor.
5. The diameter of the tumor.

In the event that there is a question as to whether or not invasion is present, and additional sectioning does not resolve the question, it is recommended that invasion not be diagnosed.

MICROSCOPIC MEASUREMENTS AND DEFINITIONS OF MEASUREMENTS

There are some problems related to vulvar superficially invasive carcinoma relevant to the method of measurement that will be used to determine the depth of invasion. All investigators concur that the deepest point of invasion is the correct deep measurement. All pathologists further agree that a calibrated microscope, using a calibrated ocular or other appropriate measurement device, is necessary to make precise and accurate measurements. Differences of opinion exist regarding where the superficial point of measurement should be made to determine the depth of invasion. A variety of methods have been presented including measurement from the surface, measurement from the granular layer, measurement from the tip of the deepest adjacent rete ridge, measurement from the tip of the deepest adjacent tumor-free rete ridge to the deepest point of invasion, and measurement from the epithelial stromal junction of the adjacent most superficial dermal papillae (Wilkinson, 1982). Of these, measurement from the surface and measurement from the epithelial stromal junction of the adjacent dermal papillae have gained general acceptance. In the case of ulceration of the surface epithelium, measurement from the surface would not reflect a true depth, but could seriously underestimate the depth of invasion. Marked hyperkeratosis could also cause underestimation. In such cases, measurement from the granular layer of the overlying epithelium is advised but would be possible only if the surface epithelium were intact and a granular layer present. Tumors arising within the vulvar vestibule may not have a granular layer because this area normally does not have a keratinized surface. Measurement from the surface, or granular layer if keratinized, to the deepest point of invasion is referred to as the *thickness of the tumor*. Measurement from the deep tip of an overlying rete ridge is unreliable because rete ridge itself is usually involved in the neoplastic process or a hyperplastic process. The same concern applies when attempting to find areas of rete ridges not involved with the overlying neoplastic process.

This could result in an incorrect underestimation of the depth of invasion.

Measurement from the epithelial stromal junction of the adjacent most superficial dermal papillae to the deepest point of invasion is referred to as the *depth of invasion* and can be found in all sites in the vulva and it will not be significantly influenced by hyperkeratosis, tumor surface ulceration, or adjacent epithelial neoplasia or hyperplasia. This measurement may not be possible in deeply invasive tumor due to their size. The International Society of Gynecological Pathologists Terminology Committee suggests that this measurement be referred to as "*the depth of invasion*" and that the measurement from the surface, or granular layer if keratin is present, be referred to as the "*thickness of the tumor*." In superficially invasive tumors, the depth of invasion method is useful; however, in more deeply invasive tumors, the tumor thickness is usually easier to measure. The major limiting factor is in dealing with cases where there is no adjacent normal skin or mucous membrane adjacent to the tumor on the side being used for measurement.

CLINICAL BEHAVIOR AND TREATMENT

With 1-mm depth of invasion the frequency of inguinal lymph node metastasis is essentially zero (Iversen et al., 1981; Wilkinson et al., 1982; Hoffman et al., 1983; Dvoretsky et al., 1984; Kneale et al., 1984; Sedis et al. 1987; Wilkinson, 1987; Wilkinson, 1991; Hacker, 1994).

In patients meeting the ISSVD criteria of stage Ia carcinoma of the vulva, recommended therapy is wide local excision of the lesion without vulvectomy. Inguinal femoral lymphadenectomy generally is not necessary in these patients. Patients with more than one invasive carcinoma, or a carcinoma exceeding 1 mm depth of invasion or 2 cm in diameter require more extensive surgical therapy, generally including wide radical local excision with 3-cm surgical margins and at least ipsilateral inguinal femoral lymphadenectomy if the tumor has a depth of invasion of over 1 mm, but not exceeding 3 mm, and the lymph nodes are clinically negative. If the superficial nodes contain metastatic tumor, pelvic lymph node radiation is needed. Midline tumors of this size require bilateral inguinal femoral lymphadenectomy. More advanced tumors generally require total or hemivulvectomy with bilateral inguinal femoral lymphadenectomy and, if these nodes contain tumor, pelvic lymph node radiation therapy.

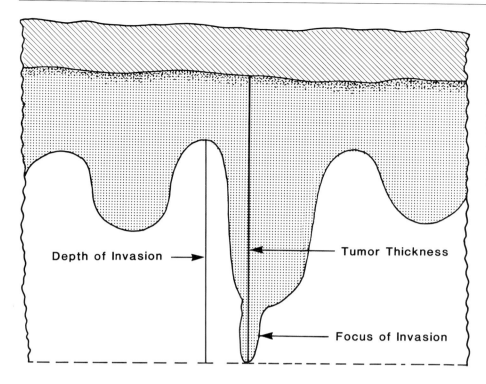

Figure 8.35. Squamous cell carcinoma. Measurements for the depth of invasion and tumor thickness. The depth of invasion is measured from the epithelial dermal junction of the adjacent dermal papillae to the deepest point of invasion. The tumor thickness is measured from the bottom of the granular zone to the deepest point of invasion or, if the epithelium is not keratinized, from the surface to the deepest point of invasion. From Wilkinson, EJ, VIN/risk of invasion. In: Damjanov I, et al. eds. Progress in Reproductive and Urinary Tract Pathology, vol. 2, New York: Field & Wood Publisher, 1990.

Depth of Invasion →

← Tumor Thickness

← Focus of Invasion

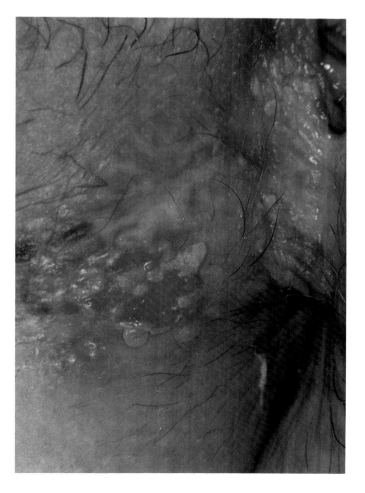

Figure 8.36. Squamous cell carcinoma. Lesion present in a patient with 9-year history of HPV/VIN. Biopsy demonstrated a 0.8-mm superficially invasive squamous cell carcinoma that was treated with wide local excision (maximum depth of invasion was 1 mm).

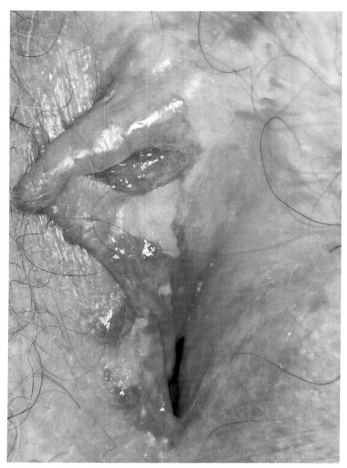

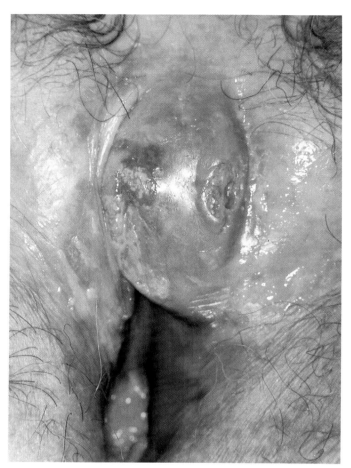

Figure 8.37. Squamous cell carcinoma. Right labial ulcer in a field of VIN and lichen sclerosus. Biopsy demonstrated squamous cell carcinoma (>2 mm invasion) and the patient underwent a modified radical right vulvectomy and partial simple left vulvectomy. Maximum depth of invasion was 3.8 mm, and 14 right inguinal nodes were negative for carcinoma.

Figure 8.38. Squamous cell carcinoma. Large ulcerating mass midline and left of the clitoris. Lesion had been present for approximately 5 months and initial biopsy had demonstrated ''inflammation.'' Failure to respond to antibiotics prompted a second biopsy, which demonstrated ''invasive squamous cell carcinoma, well-differentiated, keratinizing type.'' The patient underwent a radical vulvectomy and lymph node resection.

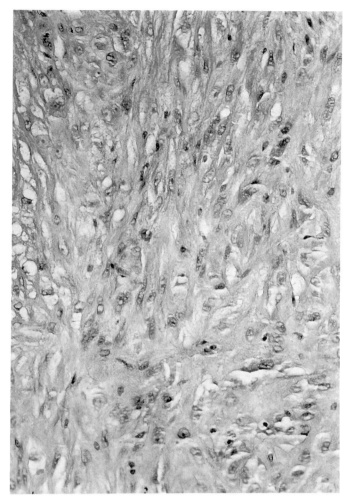

Figure 8.39. Squamous cell carcinoma, spindle cell type. The squamous cells are spindled in shape and have pleomorphic nuclei. No keratin is evident.

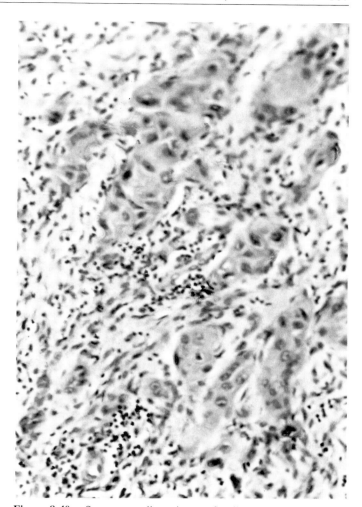

Figure 8.40. Squamous cell carcinoma. Small nests of poorly differentiated squamous cell carcinoma are seen with fibrous stroma and inflammatory cells. The tumor has a diffuse growth pattern.

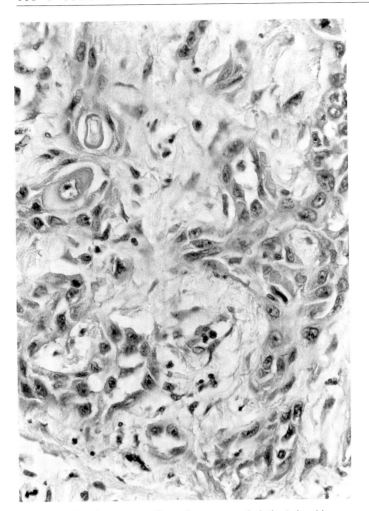

Figure 8.41. Squamous cell carcinoma, acantholytic (adenoid squamous) type. The tumor cell groups have focal central necrosis resulting in a pseudoglandular growth pattern.

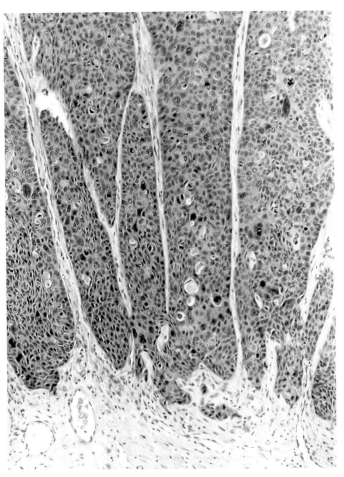

Figure 8.42. Squamous cell carcinoma. Warty VIN with warty carcinoma (condylomatous carcinoma). Focal "fingerlike" invasion is present, with neoplastic epithelium surrounded by the superficial dermis, which is desmoplastic (fibrotic) at the sites of invasion.

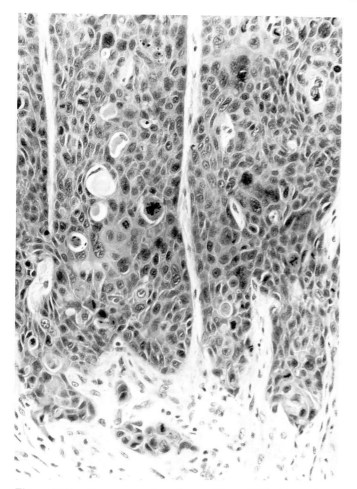

Figure 8.43. Squamous cell carcinoma. Warty VIN with condylomatous carcinoma. Higher magnification of Figure 8.40. At the tumor-dermal interface, clusters of the invasive squamous tumor can be seen in the immediately adjacent dermis. Koilocytosis and multinucleation are present.

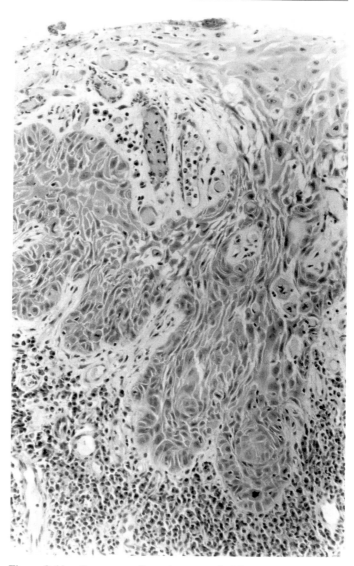

Figure 8.44. Squamous cell carcinoma, well-differentiated. The tumor is composed of well-differentiated squamous cells with prominent eosinophilic cytoplasm. The tumor has a compact of "pushing" pattern of growth in this area. Adjacent deeper tumor is illustrated in Figure 8.43.

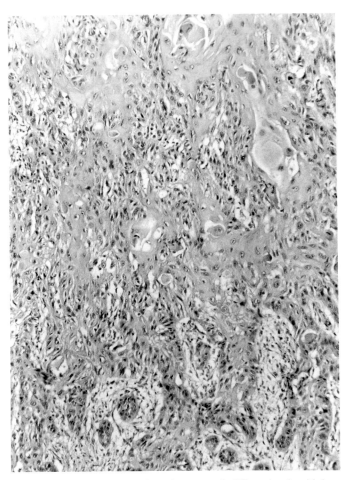

Figure 8.45. Squamous cell carcinoma, well-differentiated, with keratin formation. The tumor has cords and nests of squamous cells with prominent eosinophilic cytoplasm, moderate nuclear pleomorphism, and keratin formation. The stroma is desmoplastic and some inflammatory cells are present adjacent to the tumor.

Syphilis

DEFINITION

Syphilis is a sexually transmitted disease caused by the bacterium *Treponema pallidum*.

GENERAL FEATURES

Although present in declining numbers since the introduction of penicillin after World War II, recently the prevalence of syphilis has been increasing. There appears to be a correlation between the rise in the incidence of syphilis and the increasing prevalence of the human immunodeficiency virus in the population. Whereas it was rare to see primary or secondary syphilis in the 1970s and 1980s, increasingly patients infected with this bacterium will be seen in a busy gynecologic practice. The causative agent, *T. pallidum* is a delicate spiral organism transmitted by direct contact. The organism is extremely sensitive to drying and will not survive outside the host organism.

CLINICAL PRESENTATION

Syphilis has three distinct stages: primary, secondary, and tertiary. There are periods of latency interposed between these three stages. The first clinical evidence of infection will occur approximately 21 days after inoculation with the *Treponema* organism (range, 10–90 days). A painless ulcer will appear on the vulva, and unless palpated or visualized during self-examination, will go unnoticed in the female patient. The ulcer is sharply demarcated, hard, and usually not tender. There will usually be no purulent exudate unless the ulcer is secondarily infected. Regional lymphadenopathy is noted in the inguinal region and may be unilateral or bilateral. After 3–8 weeks the ulcer will regress and within weeks to months evidence of secondary syphilis will emerge.

Manifestations of secondary syphilis are secondary to dissemination of the *Treponema* organisms throughout the body. Systemic symptoms such as fever, arthralgias, bone pain, and malaise may be noted. Diffuse skin lesions may be present and may be annular, maculopapular, papular, or macular. Most commonly the lesions are maculopapular and frequently are found on the palms and soles, demonstrating a brownish coloration. On the genitalia, the classic lesion of secondary syphilis is condyloma lata. These lesions are teeming with *Treponema* organisms and are usually multiple, broad-based plaques with a gray-pink to white color. They may be observed in other moist regions of the body, such

as the axilla and under the breasts. Involvement of the periosteum may result in bone pain especially in the skull, clavicle, tibia, and radius. Liver involvement may present as abdominal discomfort and jaundice. Ocular involvement may present as painful reddened conjunctivitis or scleritis. Iritis may result in photophobia and visual dimness.

Late or tertiary syphilis usually will present with neurologic manifestations or cardiac manifestations secondary to gumma development within these vital structures.

The diagnosis of syphilis should be entertained in any patient with vulvar ulceration. Although the primary lesion of syphilis, the chancre, is classically firm, clean-based, well-demarcated, and not tender, secondary infection may result in a pattern suggestive of infection due to herpes or *H. ducreyi*. Both herpes and *H. ducreyi* induce skin ulcerations that typically are painful. Lymphogranuloma venereum may also be associated with vulvar ulcerations and lymphadenopathy. HIV may be associated with primary ulcerations of the vulva that are often indistinguishable from those ulcerations seen with syphilis. Dark-field or immunofluorescent examination of chancre fluid may demonstrate the characteristic spirochete. The standard diagnostic approach is to obtain dark-field or immunofluorescent examination and follow-up with serologic testing. A VDRL and RPR are qualitative and quantitative measurements of antibodies against cardiolipin. Unfortunately, these tests may be falsely positive in patients who have lupus, hepatitis, sarcoidosis, recent immunization, drug abuse, or pregnancy. Also in secondary syphilis a prozone phenomenon may be noted in which the tests are falsely negative because of the marked elevation in anticardiolipin antibody that may interfere with the test. Dilution of the serum will be necessary to assay for true activity. A more specific test for treponemal infection is the fluorescent treponemal antibody absorbed test. Nonspecific and specific serology should be obtained to evaluate vulvar ulceration. If suspicion exists for the presence of other pathogens, obtain herpes cultures, *H. ducreyi* cultures, and serologic testing for *C. trachomatis*. All patients with vulvar ulcerations suggestive of syphilis should also be counseled for HIV testing. Not only does this testing have diagnostic ramifications, it has major therapeutic ramifications, as will be discussed later.

Diagnosis of lesions of secondary syphilis will be based primarily on serologic testing. Secretions from mucocutaneous lesions may be examined under darkfield magnification. Serologic testing with the VDRL (or RPR) and fluorescent treponemal antibody test should be obtained. As with primary syphilis, HIV testing should be strongly advised. The condyloma lata lesions of secondary syphilis are often confused with condylomata acuminata and have been treated with topical agents because of an incorrect diagnosis. Failure of "condylomata acuminata" lesions to respond to topical therapy should prompt reconsideration of diagnosis and appropriate evaluation for secondary syphilis.

Patients with latent syphilis greater than 1 year in duration, tertiary syphilis, and possibly all patients who test positive for HIV should be considered for lumbar puncture. Lumbar puncture will assist in defining the presence of *T. pallidum* in the central nervous system. It should be noted that approximately 50% of patients with primary syphilis will have neurologic involvement. Before the current epidemic of HIV, neurosyphilis was rarely seen after initiating standard penicillin therapy. With the evolution of the AIDS epidemic, concern has mounted that standard regimens of penicillin are ineffective in managing syphilis and preventing neurosyphilis in the HIV-infected patient.

MICROSCOPIC FINDINGS

The primary syphilitic chancre is an ulcerated lesion with an acute and chronic inflammatory infiltrate characterized by a prominent perivascular plasma cell arteritis. Silver stains (Dieterle or Warthin Starry) for spirochetes will identify organisms about the vessels within the dermis.

SYPHILIS—CONDYLOMA LATUM

Unlike primary syphilitic chancre, condyloma lata is not ulcerated, but has hyperplastic epithelial features including marked acanthosis and hyperkeratosis. A perivascular plasma cell infiltrate is evident, mixed with chronic inflammatory cells within the dermis. Silver stains demonstrate large numbers of spirochetes within the lesion, primarily within the dermis, but also within the epithelium.

The preferable means to diagnose a primary chancre or condyloma lata is to prepare a scraping, or express fluid from the lesion, air-dry it, and employ a fluorescent conjugated antibody to the spirochete organism. An alternative method is dark-field examination of fresh fluid or scrapings. This requires great care to prevent drying and avoid false-negative findings. Both of these methods are superior to silver stains on tissue sections to identify spirochetes. *T. pallidum* is spiraled and has 6–14 coils. It mea-

sures up to 15 μm in length and 0.20 μm in diameter. Serologic studies for *T. pallidum* are indicated in all cases suspected of being syphilis. Up to 30% of women with chancres with identifiable organisms will have negative serology at the time of the initial visit.

CLINICAL BEHAVIOR AND TREATMENT

Treatment of early syphilis (primary syphilis, secondary syphilis, and latent syphilis less than 1 year in duration) has traditionally consisted of 2.4 million units of benzathine penicillin G given intramuscularly on one occasion (may be given as 1.2 million units in each buttock). For patients allergic to penicillin and who are not pregnant, doxycycline 100 mg twice a day for 14 days is an alternative regimen (or tetracycline 500 mg four times a day for 14 days). Pregnant patients allergic to penicillin may be treated with erythromycin 500 mg orally four times a day for approximately 14 days; however, this regimen has higher rates of relapse and patients should be followed closely with serology to confirm cure. Patients with late syphilis, defined as syphilis existing for more than 1 year, should receive 2.4 million units of benzathine penicillin G intramuscularly weekly for 3 weeks.

Patients with neurosyphilis should receive 2–4 million units of penicillin G intravenously every 4 hours for 10–14 days. An alternative approach is 2.4 million units of procaine penicillin G intramuscularly daily (plus probenecid 500 mg four times a day orally) for 10–14 days. This latter regimen precludes hospital admission. Optimum therapy for the HIV-infected patient who has concomitant syphilis is controversial. High relapse rates have been noted with the standard approach to therapy. Retreatment is often necessary and controversy exists concerning the optimum therapy for neurosyphilis within this subgroup of patients. Consultation with an infectious disease specialist dealing with HIV infections would be most appropriate. The suggestion exists that all patients who are positive for HIV and have syphilis should have lumbar puncture to exclude neurosyphilis. In the presence of neurosyphilis the standard would be to admit the patient and administer approximately 12 million units of penicillin G (in divided doses) intravenously each day for approximately 10 days, or to treat a patient as an outpatient, administering 2.4 million units of procaine penicillin intramuscularly every day for 10 days. Serologic evidence of relapse should prompt reinitiation of therapy.

Progressive Therapeutic Options

1. Primary syphilis, secondary syphilis, and latent syphilis of less than 1 year's duration: 2.4 million units of benzathine penicillin G intramuscularly (1.2 million units in each buttock). Alternative therapy for the patient allergic to penicillin who is *not* pregnant: doxycycline 100 mg twice a day for 14 days or tetracycline 500 mg orally four times a day for 14 days. For the patient who is allergic to penicillin and who is pregnant: erythromycin 500 mg orally four times a day for 14 days (higher rate of relapse than with standard regimes).

2. Latent syphilis (greater than 1 year): benzathine penicillin G 2.4 million units intramuscularly weekly for 3 weeks.

3. Neurosyphilis: Penicillin G 2–4 million units intravenously every 4 hours for 10–14 days or procaine penicillin G 2.4 million units daily for 10–14 days plus probenecid 500 mg four times a day).

4. For the patient with syphilis and HIV: discuss with infectious disease specialist advisability of standard lumbar puncture for all stages of syphilis and initiation of penicillin G 12 million units per day (in divided doses) intravenously for approximately 10 days, if the cerebrospinal fluid test result is positive.

NOTATION: All patients with vulvar ulcerations consistent with or suggestive of syphilis should be counseled for HIV testing.

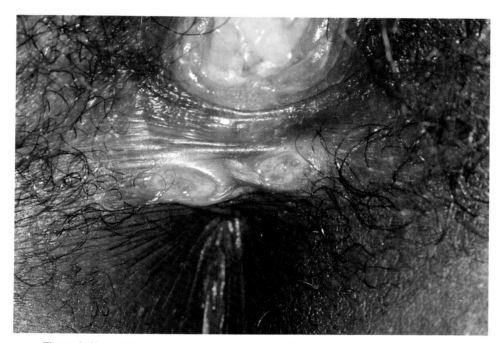

Figure 8.46. Nontender chancres ("kissing lesions") in a patient with primary syphilis.

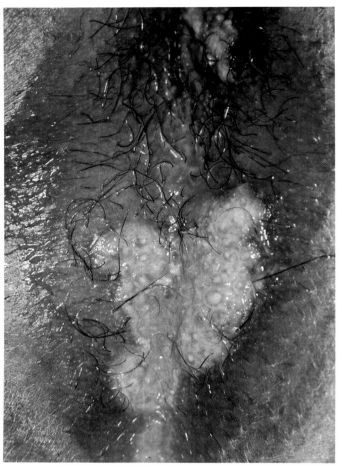

Figure 8.47. Condylomata lata in a patient with secondary syphilis. Patient had been treated with topical desiccants for presumed condylomata acuminata.

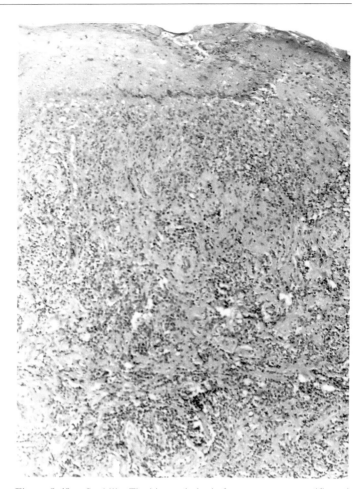

Figure 8.48. Syphilis. The histopathologic features are not specific and can vary depending upon the stage of the disease. The ulceration of the primary chancre is associated with acute and chronic inflammation within the dermis that is usually superficial and deep. Within the dermis the inflammation is primarily perivascular and associated with arteritis. Typically there are large numbers of plasma cells within the inflammatory infiltrate, which is a major clue to the diagnosis.

Systemic Lupus Erythematosus

DEFINITION

Systemic lupus erythematosus (SLE) is a connective tissue disease that affects multiple organs and is associated with antibodies to nuclear antigens.

GENERAL FEATURES

SLE is a disease more commonly seen in women than in men. There is a greater propensity for it to occur in the black population. There may be a genetic disposition for a minority of patients with the disease. Rarely, the disease may be induced by such drugs as procainamide, hydralazine, isoniazid, methyldopa, sulfonamides, and phenytoin. Oral contraceptives have been implicated in exacerbations of the disease. Exposure to sunlight may also activate the disease process. The pathogenesis of SLE involves creation of autoantibodies to DNA. The antibodies bind with antigens, creating immune complexes that adversely affect the glomeruli function, leading to renal failure. Other complexes result in a diffuse vasculitis affecting multiple organ systems.

CLINICAL PRESENTATION

Patients with SLE frequently present with a variety of cutaneous lesions, the most classic of which is the maculopapular malar rash known as the butterfly rash. A maculopapular, erythematous rash may be noted at any location on the body. Oral or vulvovaginal ulcerations may be noted in a significant number of patients, especially with a flare of the underlying systemic disease. These ulcerations may be asymptomatic or may be associated with severe discomfort. Associated with the ulcerations one may note symptoms of disease flare involving the kidneys, lungs, heart, central nervous system, gastrointestinal system, hematologic system, and joints. The flare may be so mild as to involve only the skin or so severe as to involve multiple organ failure. Usually the patient presenting with vulvovaginal ulceration will have a known diagnosis of lupus and no biopsy will be necessary for confirmation of the diagnosis. The ulcerations will involve the vestibule and vagina. They may appear as fissures and as a diffuse erythematous macular eruption involving the vaginal mucosa and vestibule. The patient presenting with such disease process and an unknown history of lupus should be evaluated for this disease entity as part of the initial workup. An antinuclear antibody should be obtained as a screen. Additional antibodies such as anti-Sm may

be very specific for patients with lupus but these antibodies are not present in the majority of patients. Complement levels may be helpful especially in patients with active lupus nephritis. C4 and C3 may be significantly depressed with active nephritis. Liver function tests may demonstrate evidence of hepatic failure. Hematologic studies may demonstrate leukopenia, anemia, and thrombocytopenia. Renal studies may manifest significant evidence of dysfunction (proteinuria, elevated blood urea nitrogen, and creatinine).

MICROSCOPIC FEATURES

Involvement of the vulvar skin may occur with either SLE or discoid (cutaneous) lupus erythematosus. Vacuolar change of the basal and parabasal keratinocytes, with the formation of intracytoplasmic vacuoles in the keratinocytes at the epidermal-dermal interface is the most distinctive feature of both systemic and discoid lupus erythematosis. In addition, both types have a lymphocytic infiltrate within the dermis, which is superficial and deep and involves perivascular as well as periinfundibular areas. Mucin within the reticular dermis may be seen in both forms, but is more pronounced in SLE. Involvement of the underyling fat is an important feature characterizing lupus. Lymphocytes can be found in the superficial intralobular areas of the adjacent adipose tissue. The cell wall of adipocytes also may be thickened and basophilic.

In SLE, the epithelium is typically not significantly altered; however, in discoid lupus erythematosus, the epithelium may be significantly changed, ranging from markedly thickened and acanthotic to thinned and atrophic. Hyperkeratosis is usually present, but is not a consistent finding. The keratinocyte vacuolar change may be striking with associated dyskeratosis and colloid bodies.

Immunofluorescent studies (lupus band test) for IgG, IgM, and complement may be complementary in SLE, where granular deposits are usually seen of one or all of these components. The deposits are not identified in discoid lupus erythematosus; however, immunofluorescent studies are not considered totally reliable in distinguishing these two forms of lupus erythematosus.

ADJUNCTIVE STUDIES

No adjunctive studies are necessary in patients with a known history of lupus other than definition of the current status of various organs potentially involved by the disease.

DIFFERENTIAL DIAGNOSIS

The differential diagnosis of vulvovaginal ulceration in a patient with known lupus is limited. The disease state is fairly characteristic; however, any ulcerative process may account for disease and should be entertained in the differential diagnosis. The sexually active patient with vulvar ulcerations may be suffering from herpes and the patient's immune status may be significantly impaired if she is being currently managed with steroids to control her SLE. Ulcerations associated with HSV are painful and are preceded by a vesicular eruption. The patient should be queried concerning her sexual history and any history of herpes infection. Appropriate cultures should be obtained for herpes if uncertainty exists concerning the diagnosis. The sexually active patient may also be at risk for syphilis; however, syphilis is not a diffuse process involving the vagina and vulva and would rarely be confused with lupus. Behcet's disease is also a vasculitis that may present with systemic manifestations and vulvar and oral ulcerations. There is not typically erythematous involvement of the vagina in Behcet's disease and this may be a helpful differential. The ulcers in Behcet's disease may be deeply seated in the vulvar region and this is not characteristically seen with lupus. Lupus ulcerations are more superficial. The antinuclear antibody is not elevated in Behcet's syndrome. Patients with AIDS may present with an ulcerative process involving the vulva and vagina. The vaginal component may be a hemorrhagic process. Immunologic compromise may result in aphthous ulcers in the mouth. Serologic screening for HIV should clarify the diagnosis.

CLINICAL BEHAVIOR AND TREATMENT

Vulvovaginal ulcerations may be directly related to disease activity and with improvement in the multisystem disease the genital process will usually improve. This will usually require increased dosages of steroids to ameliorate the systemic disease activity. While awaiting the onset of action of oral or intravenous steroids, the patient may benefit from sitz baths in Burow's solution. Failure of systemic steroids to control the genital process may require augmentation of therapy with immunosuppressant agents such as Dapsone or azathioprine (Imuran) and antimalarial drugs such as hydroxychloroquine. Other alternatives include thalidomide and isotretionin. All of these potential immunosuppressant or augmentative pharmacologic agents should be used in concert with the primary physician managing the systemic lupus. Renal insufficiency may require dose adjustments and should be managed by those familiar with the pharmacokinetics of immunosuppressants in such conditions.

Progressive Therapeutic Options

1. Increase maintenance steroid dose by administering pulse therapy, either intravenously or orally. Oral therapy may require 30–60 mg of prednisone for initial control and based upon response a rapid taper to a higher maintenance dose may be accomplished.
2. Dapsone may be administered at 50–100 mg per day. Before administering Dapsone a G6PD screen should be obtained and if normal the medication may be prescribed; however weekly complete blood cell counts should be obtained. The medication should be discontinued if anemia occurs. Dapsone should not be administered to patients with a G6PD deficiency. Dapsone may be associated with motor neuropathy and should be discontinued if such occurrence is noted.
3. Antimalarial agents such as hydroxychloroquine (Plaquenil) at 400 mg once or twice daily may be used. For prolonged maintenance therapy, a small dose, (200–400 mg daily) may be prescribed. Hydroxychloroquine may be associated with reversible retinal damage. Baseline and periodic (every 3 months) ophthalmologic examinations should be performed. Alterations in visual acuity or visual fields, or any visual symptoms should prompt discontinuation of the medication; however, retinal changes may progress after cessation of therapy.

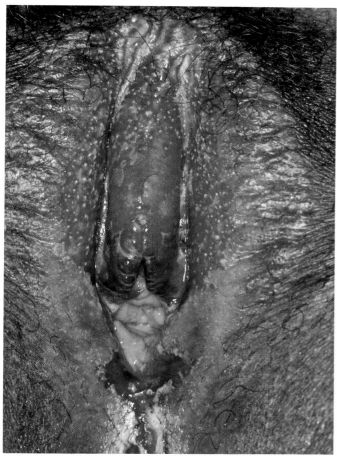

Figure 8.49. Painful vulvar (and vaginal) ulcers and fissures in a patient with known SLE. The lesions are also present in the patient's mouth.

Vulvar Crohn's Disease

DEFINITION

Crohn's disease is a chronic, noncaseating granulomatous disease that primarily affects bowel but which may present with significant vulvar and perineal involvement. The etiology of Crohn's disease is presently unknown.

CLINICAL PRESENTATION

Crohn's disease of the vulva is a rare condition that can occur in children and adults. It is usually associated with concomitant inflammatory disease of the bowel, most commonly involving the distal ileum and colon. Rarely, vulvar disease may antecede manifestations of bowel disease. Vulvar Crohn's disease may be contiguous with inflammatory bowel pathology or may be metastatic. In the latter form of Crohn's disease, no communication is noted between the vulvar lesions and the bowel lesions. Hence, in the patient with metastatic Crohn's disease, there may be no suspicion of bowel involvement if vulvar symptoms precede bowel symptoms. Most patients with vulvar Crohn's disease will present with ulcerations of the vulva that have a characteristic "knifelike" appearance. These ulcerations appear in the folds of the vulva, occurring between the labia majora and the medial thighs or between the labia minora and the labia majora. They may progress to deep-seated ulcers. Pain associated with them may limit the patient's mobility and intercourse may become impossible. Although these ulcers may appear to be infected, and the sinus tracts may drain watery fluid resembling small bowel contents, the condition appears to be primarily inflammatory and patients do not typically present with evidence of sepsis.

The diagnosis of Crohn's disease of the vulva must be entertained in patients presenting with the classic "knifelike" ulcerations at skin folds. These are considered pathognomonic of vulvar Crohn's disease. Vulvar ulcerations in patients with known bowel involvement with Crohn's disease usually may be attributed to the primary granulomatous disease without extensive evaluation.

MICROSCOPIC FEATURES

The characteristic histopathologic findings in vulvar Crohn's disease include noncaseating granulomatous inflammation involving both the superficial and deep dermis. The ulcerated surface and sinus tracts, if present, are associated with granulation tissue which is especially prominent about the edges of the ulcer. Stains for fungi, acid-fast bacteria, spirochetes, and bacteria do not demonstrate organisms.

DIFFERENTIAL DIAGNOSIS

Other diseases to be considered in the differential diagnosis include hidradenitis suppurativa, lymphogranuloma venereum, Behcet's disease and tuberculosis. Biopsy may be necessary to define the etiology of the ulcerative process. In addition, radiographic and endoscopic bowel evaluation may be necessary to assess for inflammatory disease in the patient with vulvar involvement but no symptoms of bowel disease.

CLINICAL BEHAVIOR AND TREATMENT

Crohn's disease is a chronic inflammatory process that clinically may wax and wane over many years. For mild vulvar disease, topical applications of steroids may be effective; however, most patients will require the initiation of systemic therapy. Metronidazole has demonstrated efficacy in controlling the clinical manifestations of vulvar Crohn's disease. Metronidazole may be commenced at an oral dose of 250–500 mg three times a day. This dose may be adjusted up or down based upon the clinical response. It will be necessary to maintain this therapy, usually for several months at the lower dose of 250 mg taken three times daily. Patients should be cautioned that peripheral neuropathy may develop and seizures have been noted on long-term metronidazole therapy. Patients with a history of such neurologic problems should be monitored closely and alternative therapy should be considered. Patients who are taking metronidazole should be forewarned that consumption of alcohol may induce nausea and emesis. Periodic assessment of white blood cell and platelet counts should be obtained to rule out glanulocytopenia or thrombocytopenia, which may occur on long-term metronidazole therapy.

Oral prednisone frequently will be required to control disease activity. Low-dose maintenance therapy may be used during periods of relative inactivity; however, a marked exacerbation of disease will require bursts of high-dose steroids, typically prednisone 60 mg/day with a slow taper over succeeding weeks as disease activity diminishes. Exacerbation of the Crohn's disease will require strict vulvar hygiene and is most easily accomplished with whirlpool baths. Daily whirlpool baths are soothing and appear to augment the healing process.

In the patient with recalcitrant disease and minimal amelioration with high-dose steroid therapy and maximum metronidazole therapy, consideration should be given to initiation of azathioprine (Imuran) immunosuppression. This medication may be initiated at a dose of 1 mg/kg/day. After 6 weeks, if no untoward toxicity is noted and there appears to be no clinical response, the dose may be increased to 2 mg/kg/day with close monitoring of blood parameters. Parameters to be followed include complete blood cell count, liver function tests, and lipase and amylase levels. The rarity of vulvar Crohn's disease has precluded controlled studies supporting the use of immunosuppressant therapy; however, there is the observation in inflammatory bowel disease that immunosuppressant therapy may be beneficial in managing this disabling condition.

The patient for whom pharmacologic therapy fails becomes a candidate for surgical excision of the Crohn's disease. Most commonly, surgical therapy will consist of wide local excision. Healing may be delayed, especially in the patient who has been managed with chronic steroid therapy. The excision is much the same as is used to treat patients with hidradenitis suppurativa. Frequently, the patient with vulvar Crohn's disease undergoing partial vulvectomy will have had an antecedent diverting procedure for bowel involvement; therefore, less soilage of the operative field postoperatively is expected with the diversion in place.

Progressive Therapeutic Options

1. Oral metronidazole at 250–500 mg three times a day with dose adjusted up or down based on clinical response (long-term therapy will be necessary).
2. Oral prednisone:
   (a) minor disease activity: 5 mg every day or every other day.
   (b) acute exacerbation: 60 mg every day followed by taper.
3. For recalcitrant disease consider azathioprine 1–2 kg/day (monitor complete blood cell count, liver function tests, amylase, lipase).
4. With failed pharmacologic intervention, wide excision should be considered.

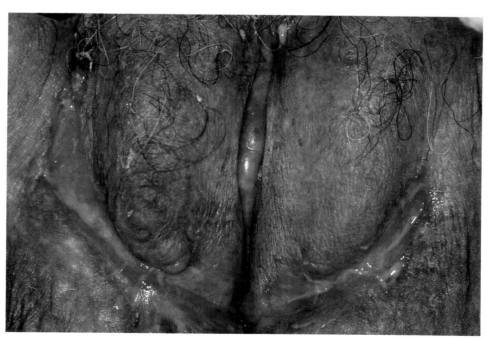

Figure 8.50. Classic "knifelike" ulcerations in a patient with vulvar Crohn's disease.

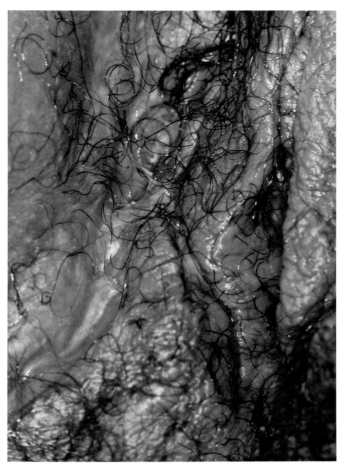

Figure 8.51. Deep vulvar ulceration in a patient with Crohn's disease of the vulva and bowel for approximately 9 years. Exacerbation of vulvar disease was unresponsive to prednisone 60 mg orally every day and metronidazole 500 mg orally three times a day. Imuran was started at 100 mg orally every day.

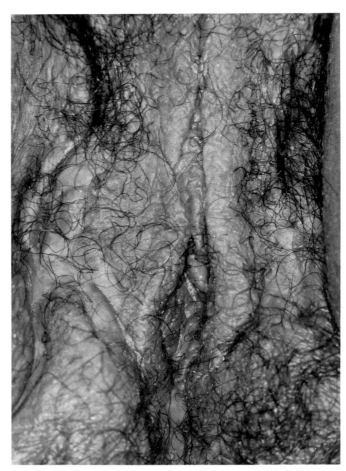

Figure 8.52. Patient in Figure 8.49 after approximately 8 weeks of Imuran and prednisone.

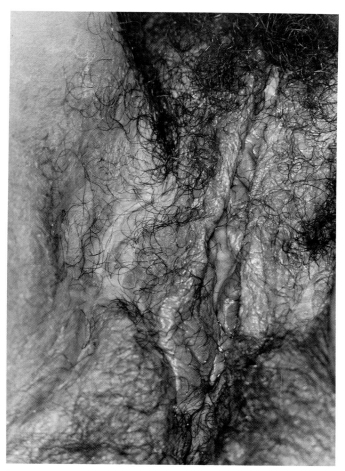

Figure 8.53. Patient in Figure 8.49 after approximately 12 weeks of Imuran and prednisone. Ulcer has healed. Prednisone taper has commenced. Complete response has lasted 14 months on Imuran.

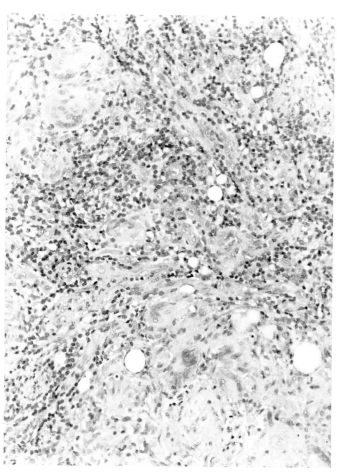

Figure 8.54. Crohn's disease. Ulceration with fistula formation is present. The chronic inflammatory infiltrate is superficial and deep and associated with noncaseating granulomas. Organisms are not identified.

$\mathcal{9}$

VERRUCAE

VERRUCA ALGORITHM

VERRUCA (Latin verruca: wart): a lobulated, hyperplastic lesion with a horny surface.

Description	Presumed diagnosis
Multifocal	Condylomata acuminata
Unifocal	Condyloma acuminatum
	Verrucous carcinoma

Figure 9.1. Verruca algorithm.

Condyloma Acuminatum

DEFINITION

A verrucous lesion characterized by acanthosis with elongation and thickening of the rete ridges, usually displaying cytopathic effects caused by human papillomavirus (HPV) infection.

GENERAL FEATURES

The terminology condyloma acuminatum is derived from the Greek phrase for a caruncle or node and the Latin phrase for sharply pointed. This derivation accurately describes the most common sexually transmitted disease seen by obstetricians and gynecologists in the 1990s. Induced by the human papillomavirus, the resultant warty growths in the lower reproductive tract have become a major nuisance for the patient and a therapeutic nightmare for the physician. Unfortunately, what begins as a nuisance may evolve into a life-threatening condition, especially if the initiating organism is a type 16 or type 18 human papillomavirus. There is particular concern that these types have a proclivity to induce dysplastic and neoplastic changes in the lower reproductive tract. Although other types have been observed in dysplastic and neoplastic lesions, types 16 and 18 are by far the most frequently observed types in dysplastic lesions. Extremely specific and sensitive polymerase-chain reaction studies indicate that human papillomavirus has widespread prevalence in the general population. Although the incubation period for human papillomavirus is noted to be approximately 3 months, the inability to study the virus in an animal model has resulted in poorly understood epidemiology. It is possible that incubation periods may be vastly underestimated. Subclinical infection with human papillomavirus may be present for months to years before clinical evidence of the disease becomes manifest.

CLINICAL PRESENTATION

Patients with clinical disease will present complaining of warty growths on the vulvar skin. They may have been present for variable periods of time and occasionally a patient will wait months before presenting for evaluation. On examination the typical verrucous, papillary lesions will be noted on the vulvar skin. Commonly, multiple lesions will be noted. The lesions may be observed on the vestibule, the labia minora, the labia majora, and the perianal regions. Examination of the vagina will frequently demonstrate disease in the vagina and on the cervix. Approximately 40–50% of patients with vulvar disease will have evidence of human papillomavirus on the cervix. Disease is especially widespread in immunosuppressed, transplant, diabetic, autoimmune, and AIDS patients. Frequently in immunosuppressed patients evidence of viral disease will be noted elsewhere, such as on the extremities, where common warts may be noted. Excessive growth of the verrucous lesions may impair the patient's ability to have vaginal intercourse. Maintenance of proper hygiene after defecation may become impossible.

The diagnosis of condylomata acuminata is most frequently made by visual inspection. The classic warty growths are well known to clinicians. Rarely is it necessary to biopsy such lesions. Small unifocal lesions may be confused with skin tags or intradermal nevi. More diffuse lesions rarely may be confused with condyloma lata, vulvar intraepithelial neoplasia, and verrucous carcinoma. When uncertainty exists, or when therapeutic intervention fails to ameliorate the condition, biopsy should be performed for a confirmation of diagnosis. The clinical usefulness of HPV serotyping has not been documented and is currently not cost-effective. Regardless of the human papilloma serotype involved, patients should be observed closely for evidence of dysplastic or neoplastic growth on a long-term basis.

MICROSCOPIC FINDINGS

The histopathologic findings in vulvar condyloma acuminatum can be highly variable depending upon the age of the lesion, prior or current therapy, and location on the vulva. Vulvar condylomata acuminata may vary considerably in size and in growth pattern from relatively flat and papular to markedly verrucoid and papillomatous. Microscopic features include parabasalar hyperplasia, accentuation of intracellular bridges, koilocytosis, dyskeratosis, hyperkeratosis, and parakeratosis. Condylomata involving the vulvar vestibule usually are not hyperkeratotic and may be relatively flat with prominent koilocytosis and multinucleated keratinocytes. On the hairy keratinized skin of the vulva, condylomata may have a prominent granular layer with a verrucoid structure. In skin areas, koilocytes may be rare, and present only in focal areas. Unlike vulvar intrathelial neoplasia, the keratinocytes of condylomata have relatively uniform nuclei with vesicular chromatin, and lack hyperchromasia. Mitotic figures, when present, are in the basal and parabasal areas, and are not atypical. If the patient has had topical podophyllin applied within 1–2 weeks of biopsy, mitotic figures may be prevalent and may be abnormal in appearance. Because of this, it is usu-

ally advisable to wait at least 2 weeks after discontinuing podophyllin before biopsy of the condylomata.

Occasionally, condylomata acuminata of the vulva are pigmented. In these cases, melanin is found in the basal cells as well as within some of the keratinocytes of the condyloma. Melanin-laden dermal macrophages may be evident. Clinically, pigmented condylomata may be mistaken for pigmented vulvar intrathelial neoplasia, seborrheic keratosis, or nevomelanocytic lesions.

CLINICAL BEHAVIOR AND TREATMENT

Small unifocal or multifocal lesions may be easily treated in the clinic setting with application of bichloroacetic or trichloroacetic acid. This desiccant therapy is quite effective in managing small lesions. It must be remembered that the normal-appearing vulvar skin is quite sensitive to these desiccants and the liquid should be applied primarily to the wart and a small margin of surrounding skin. To prevent spread of the caustic agent to other areas, petroleum jelly may be applied to the skin surrounding the wart before application of the chemical. Application of desiccant is quite painful and the patient should be forewarned that discomfort will be transient but significant. Bichloroacetic acid and trichloroacetic acid are not known to be embryotoxic or teratogenic and therefore can be used on the vulva during pregnancy. This cannot be said for the podophyllin derivatives, where concern for inducing adverse fetal effects precludes their use in pregnancy. Frequently it is not known whether the patient is pregnant and use of chloroacetic acid does not necessitate a pretherapy pregnancy test. Recently, a podophyllin derivative, podofilox, has become available for home use. Whereas trichloroacetic acid applications require return visits at 1–2 week intervals until the entire wart has been desiccated, 0.5% podofilox solution may be applied at home by the patient. The solution is applied to the genital warts for 3 consecutive days followed by 4 drug-free days, through 4 cycles. As with the use of trichloroacetic acid, podofilox is most efficacious with smaller lesions. Larger lesions may be excised in the clinic, if they are pedunculated. Large sessile lesions pose difficulty and are best managed with laser vaporization. Office excision is accomplished under local anesthesia. The loop electrical excision device may be used to excise condylomata in the office setting under appropriate local anesthesia. Electrical grounding is mandatory. The patient and health care providers should wear viral protective face masks and the generated plume should be evacuated by suction.

Multifocal disease is most appropriately managed with laser therapy. This will require regional or general anesthesia in the operating room. Extensive evaluation before use of the laser should define the extent of the disease. This will require colposcopic examination after application of 3–5% acetic acid to the vulva. Subclinical regions of human papillomavirus infection will appear white under colposcopic examination and should be included in the laser ablation. Attention should be paid to the vagina and cervix before operating room intervention. Significant involvement of the cervix with human papillomavirus or with a dysplastic process may require operative management. Care should be taken during the ablation of the condylomata to evacuate the plume, and health care providers should wear appropriate masks to prevent inhalation of viral particles. The condylomata should be lasered to the first surgical plane of the epidermis in the nonpilosebaceous regions. In the pilosebaceous regions the laser ablation will be most efficacious if it is taken to the second surgical plane just above the reticular dermis, where a typical yellowish coloration is noted during laser ablation. Deeper ablation in the pilosebaceous region is necessary to destroy virus residing in pilosebaceous ducts and glands. Close attention should be paid to the urethra and the anus. Persistent disease in these two areas may serve as a nidus for recurrence of condylomata after surgical ablation. If the perianal region is ablated, a moist sponge should be placed in the anus to prevent explosion of bowel gas and resultant tissue injury. Power densities should be in the range of 750 watts for laser ablation of condylomata. Bleeding may be controlled by defocusing the laser. Brush laser of the surrounding vulvar skin should be accomplished. This will theoretically destroy virus residing in normal-appearing epithelium. This may be accomplished by placing the laser on superpulse and moving the wand back and forth in a rapid motion. The skin will bubble and will be easily desquamated with a moist sponge. Periodic cooling of the vulva should be accomplished with cold soaks during laser ablation. After surgery, Silvadene may be applied to the vulva, and oral analgesics usually will be necessary.

Extensive disease, especially in immunocompromised patients, may benefit from postlaser augmentation with interferon injections for 8–10 weeks. Interferon injections may be initiated intraoperatively and may be repeated Mondays, Wednesdays, and Fridays or alternatively may be used on Tuesdays and Thursdays, based upon the particular interferon being used. Interferon α-2b (intron A) may be administered intradermally (3 million IU) on Mondays, Wednesdays, and Fridays for 8 weeks. Although interferon injections may be efficacious as sole therapy for condylomata acuminata, cost-effectiveness may preclude their use for small lesions. Large, multiple lesions are most easily managed with laser therapy.

For the markedly immunocompromised patient who has received laser ablation and who has commenced interferon prophylaxis, an additional consideration is application of 5% 5-fluorouracil to the vulvar skin after healing of the laser bed is noted. It is important to note that 5% 5-fluorouracil should not be used in pregnant patients or patients who are involved in unprotected intercourse. The topical agent will cause intense reaction of vulvar skin, but may be used once or twice daily to augment the response of laser therapy. Long term use of 5% 5-fluorouracil may reduce recurrence of condylomata after healing has been observed after laser ablation. The cream may be applied to the vulva every 2 weeks for several months after surgery. Patient acceptance will be based upon the degree of inflammatory response noted.

The patient with condylomata acuminata should be warned that the disease is extremely difficult to eradicate. Laser ablation is by no means a guarantee of long-term suppression. It is impossible to eradicate the virus from the immunosuppressed patient and it may be necessary to return periodically to the operating room to ablate extensive condylomata acuminata that are becoming symptomatic and interfering with the patient's normal lifestyle. Whether recurrent disease is evidence of persistent human papillomavirus or whether it represents reacquisition through sexual contact often will be difficult to discern. The efficacy of barrier contraception for preventing acquisition of human papillomavirus is uncertain. Long-term follow-up and close observation for development of recurrent disease, with special attention to the development of cervical dysplasia, are mandatory. Persistent disease should be biopsied to rule out dysplasia. Areas that appear ulcerative or suggestive of an invasive process should be biopsied before any effort to ablate by laser. Invasive disease is not treated with the laser.

Progressive Therapeutic Options

1. For small lesions apply trichloroacetic or bichloroacetic acid focally to the lesion and a small surrounding margin of normal skin. The patient should return at weekly intervals for reapplication until desiccation of the lesion or lesions has been accomplished.
2. For the patient with small lesions who wishes to attempt self-treatment at home, podofilox solution may be applied for 3 days of therapy followed by 4 days of abstinence, repeated for a total of 4 cycles. The solution is applied twice daily with a cotton tip applicator and no more than 0.5 mL of solution should be applied per day. This substance should not be used in pregnant patients.
3. For patients with extensive disease, laser ablation offers the greatest chance for successful amelioration. Laser ablation is most commonly accomplished in the operating room under appropriate general or regional anesthesia. Not only should the obvious condylomata acuminata be ablated, but brush lasering should be done of normal, surrounding vulvar skin to decrease the risk of recurrence. Careful attention should be paid to lesons involving the urethra and anus. Ablation should be accomplished in these regions if colposcopic or gross evidence of disease is apparent. A moistened sponge should be placed in the anus to prevent explosions induced by laser contact with bowel gas. Laser ablation should be accomplished to the first surgical plane (second surgical plane in the pilosebaceous region) to decrease risk of recurrence. Postoperative application of Silvadene should be advised.
4. For the immunosuppressed patient or the patient with recalcitrant condylomata acuminata, laser ablation may be augmented with postoperative administration of interferon for 8–10 weeks injected into the vulvar skin. Additional augmentation of response may be accomplished by topical application of 5% 5-fluorouracil to the vulva once or twice daily for 3–4 weeks after healing of the laser bed has been observed. Duration of therapy will be based upon the patient's ability to withstand the caustic reaction occurring after application of 5% 5-fluorouracil.
5. Long-term prophylaxis against recalcitrant condylomata acuminata may be attempted in the patient who is not pregnant and who is using optimum birth control with the application of 5% 5-fluorouracil to the vulva every 2 weeks. If the patient cannot assure adequate contraception, then 5% 5-fluorouracil should not be administered because it may be teratogenic or embryotoxic.
6. Persistent disease unresponsive to pharmacologic intervention or surgical intervention requires biopsy to rule out vulvar intraepithelial neoplasia or carcinoma. Unusual lesions should likewise be biopsied before initiating any therapy. Increasing prevalence of syphilis will result in larger numbers of patients with condylomata lata, which are frequently confused with condylomata acuminata. Appropriate biopsies, darkfield examination, and serologic studies are mandated.

NOTATION: Patients with recurrent or persistent extensive disease should be candidates for human immunodeficiency virus screening, diabetes screening, and screening for autoimmune disease, such as lupus.

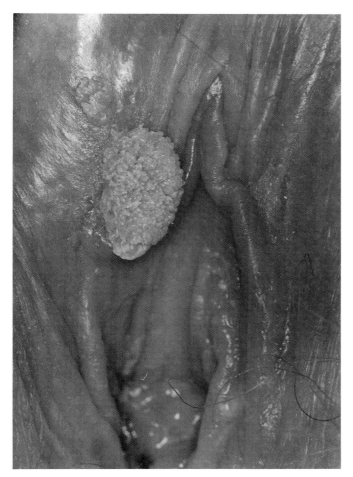

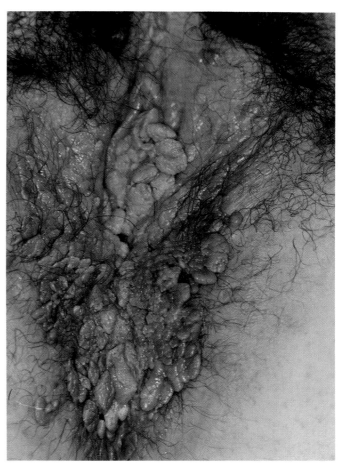

Figure 9.2. Recurrent condyloma in a nonimmunosuppressed patient previously treated with podophyllin, 5% 5-fluorouracil, electrocoagulation, and two applications of laser ablation. The condyloma was managed with excision and a course of interferon with recurrence.

Figure 9.3. Extensive vulvar condylomata acuminata in a patient managed with laser ablation.

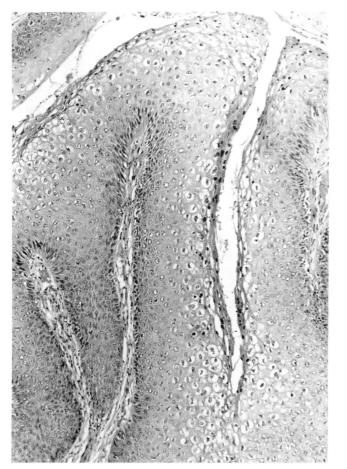

Figure 9.4. Condyloma acuminatum. The epithelial surface is verrucoid and the epithelium is thickened and acanthous. Some lack of cellular maturation is evident. A few cells near the surface have koilocytosis. There is mild superficial chronic inflammation in the dermis.

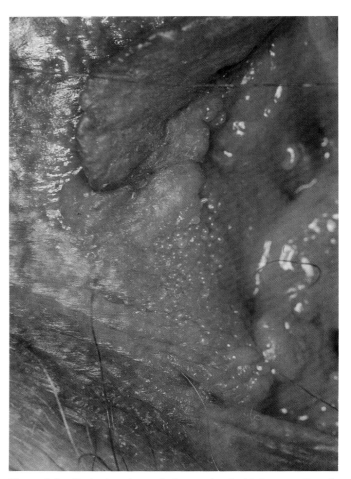

Figure 9.5. Projections in vestibule associated with long-standing discomfort, unresponsive to steroid injections and creams. Biopsy was consistent with condylomata acuminata.

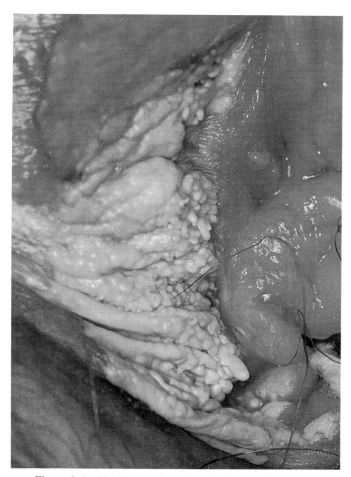

Figure 9.6. Trichloroacetic acid applied to vestibular HPV.

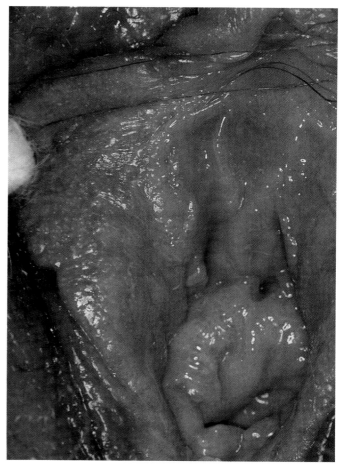

Figure 9.7. Four weeks after application of trichloroacetic acid, condylomata have resolved. With complete healing, discomfort has resolved.

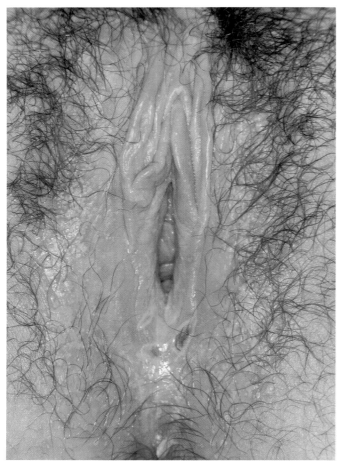

Figure 9.8. Aceto-white epithelium in a patient unresponsive to laser, Condylox, and 5% 5-fluorouracil.

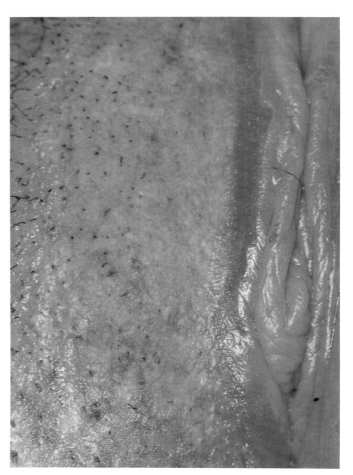

Figure 9.9. Laser ablation through first and to second surgical plane of the patient in Figure 9.8. A Sharplan Swiftlase laser was used.

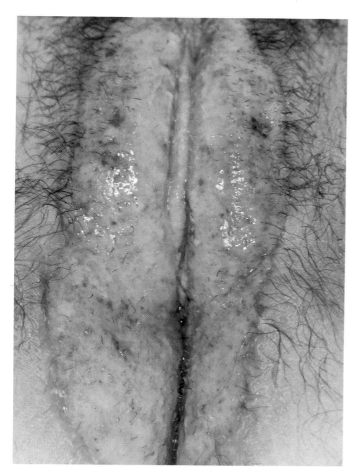

Figure 9.10. Inflammatory reaction noted 4 days after laser application at commencement of interferon augmentation.

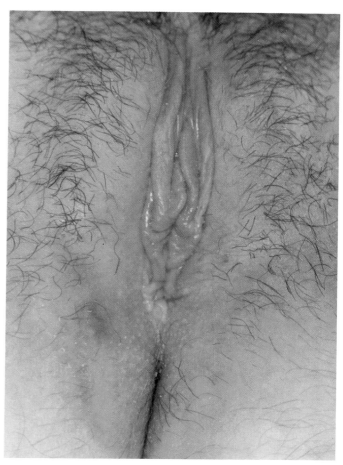

Figure 9.11. Vulva at completion of interferon injections 10 weeks after laser ablation. Colposcopic examination demonstrates no aceto-white epithelium.

Verrucous Carcinoma

DEFINITION

Verrucous carcinoma is a well-differentiated squamous carcinoma exhibiting a verrucous pattern and only local invasion. A synonymous term is giant condyloma of Buschke-Löwenstein.

GENERAL FEATURES

Verrucous carcinoma is a rare, locally invasive carcinoma that is usually seen in older people.

CLINICAL PRESENTATION

The patient will usually present complaining of a mass on the vulva. The pressure phenomenon is a source of discomfort. On examination there will be a sessile mass protruding from the vulva that may encompass the entire vulva.

MICROSCOPIC FEATURES

The surface of the neoplasm is typically exophytic and may appear papillary. On cross-section, the neoplasm may be several centimeters thick, but have well-defined deep and lateral margins.

Verrucous carcinoma is characterized microscopically by a very well differentiated epithelial neoplasm. The tumor has a characteristic pushing border, where the neoplastic bullous rete extend into the underlying dermis without cellular differentiation or fingerlike growth. The bulbous epithelial growth is not separated by fibrovascular dermal papillae, or dermal cores, as is seen with acanthotic squamous epithelium or warty carcinoma. The nuclear features of the tumor demonstrate minimal nuclear pleomorphism; however, the chromatin is coarse, and various sizes of nucleoli are usually seen. Mitoses are not prominent and when seen, typically appear normal. The cytoplasm is prominent; however, dyskeratosis is usually absent. A keratinized surface with parakeratosis is common.

Verrucous carcinoma is distinguished from warty carcinoma (condylomatous carcinoma) by the presence of typical squamous carcinoma found with warty carcinoma. In addition, warty carcinoma has prominent fibrovascular cores in the papillary projections of the verrucoid portion of the tumor.

ADJUNCTIVE STUDIES

No adjunctive studies are required other than the biopsy, which must be significantly large to provide the pathologist with adequate tissue and epithelium to discern the etiology of the process. Human papillomavirus has been identified associated with verrucous carcinoma. Variants of HPV type 6 have been most commonly observed.

DIFFERENTIAL DIAGNOSIS

The diagnoses to be considered in the differential are condylomata acuminata and squamous cell carcinoma. Both of these may be excluded by biopsy.

CLINICAL BEHAVIOR AND TREATMENT

Verrucous carcinoma is a locally invasive carcinoma and does not metastasize. It is removed by wide and deep local excision and, depending upon the size of the lesion, may be removed in the clinic under local anesthesia. There is a tendency for local recurrence, which may be managed by local excision. Large lesions may require excision in the operating room.

Progressive Therapeutic Options

1. Wide local excision.

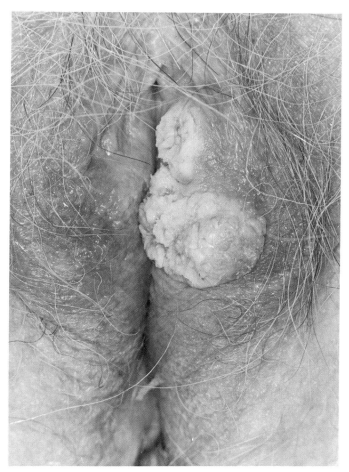

Figure 9.12. Verrucous carcinoma in an 83-year-old patient. Lesion was excised in clinic under local anesthesia. Pathology review demonstrates maximum depth of invasion to be 1 mm.

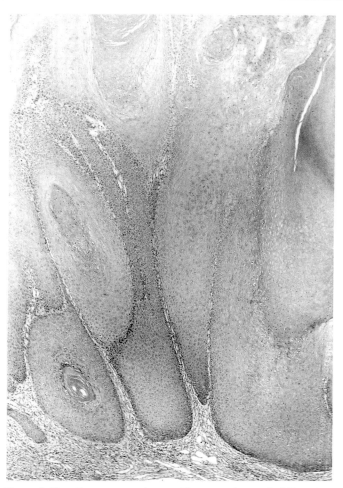

Figure 9.13. Verrucous carcinoma. The tumor is a well-differentiated squamous neoplasm with a neoplastic epithelial surface that is markedly thickened and acanthotic. The tumor has a well-defined "pushing" appearance at the dermal interface.

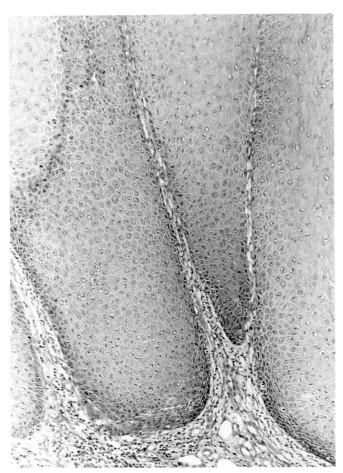

Figure 9.14. Verrucous carcinoma. Higher magnification of the adjacent field. The well-differentiated keratinocytes of the tumor have relatively dense growth, but have some maturation. The keratinocytes have prominent eosinophilic cytoplasm and nuclei with vesicular chromatin. The palisade orientation of the keratinocytes along the basement membrane is maintained, without "fingerlike" infiltrative growth. The rounded, acanthotic appearance of the invasive epithelium is evident.

10

VESICLES

(see Table A.2)

VESICLE ALGORITHM

VESICLE (Latin vesica: bladder): an epidermal
elevation, less than 0.5 cm in diameter,
containing clear fluid

Lymphangioma circumscriptum

Herpes simplex virus infection

Chickenpox (shingles)

Figure 10.1. Vesicle algorithm, excluding dermatoses. (see Table A.2)

Lymphangioma Circumscriptum

DEFINITION

Lymphangioma circumscriptum is a dilation of lymphatic channels resulting in localized vesicles.

GENERAL FEATURES

Lymphangioma circumscriptum is extremely rare. Typically the condition occurs after prior irradiation to the lower abdomen for a gynecologic malignancy. Radiation fibrosis results in obstruction in lymphatic drainage with subsequent dilation of lymph channels and the eventual eruption of vesicles on the vulvar skin. The condition may occur without prior radiation exposure but this is quite unusual.

CLINICAL PRESENTATION

The patient will present usually giving a history of prior radiation treatment. She will complain of weeping "blisters" on the vulvar skin. The loss of fluid may be extensive enough to require wearing a pad and changing the pad over the course of the day. On examination small vesicles will be noted in the pilosebaceous region of the vulva. There will often be evidence of fibrosis in the region of the mons where a radiation portal had been located previously.

MICROSCOPIC FINDINGS

The primary histologic features consist of multiple, thin-walled, endothelial lined vascular spaces that do not contain red blood cells but rather have acellular eosinophilic lymph. These vascular spaces are most prominent within the superficial papillary dermis but may also be found in the reticular dermis. These vascular structures may abut the overlying epithelium. The overlying epithelium may be slightly hyperkeratotic or within normal limits. Smooth muscle walled, dilated lymphatic vessels may be found within the immediately adjacent deeper dermis. This lesion is distinguished from angiokeratoma and superficial hemangiomas in that the vascular channels do not contain red blood cells.

DIFFERENTIAL DIAGNOSIS

Observing the vesicles on the vulvar skin would raise a suspicion of herpes. The vesicles of lymphangioma circumscriptum will have been long standing, and herpes is generally a self-limiting disease. Only in immunocompromised patients would herpetic infections result in prolonged lesions, which would usually present as ulcers rather than vesicles (see Chapter 8 for herpesvirus).

CLINICAL BEHAVIOR AND TREATMENT

Without treatment the patient can expect to have continued drainage of the vesicles. If the patient wishes to have this corrected, an option would be laser ablation of the vesicles with a CO_2 laser. The goals of laser treatment are to destroy the vesicles and to seal superficial lymphatics. Magnification should be considered when attempting to ablate the process with a CO_2 laser. An effort should be made to seal the base of the vesicles and the lymphatic channels supplying the region. An alternative approach to the CO_2 laser is the use of the flash-lamp pumped laser to destroy the vesicles. The lymphangioma circumscriptum must contain a significant hemorrhagic component to permit absorption of the emitted light by oxyhemoglobin. Although this form of laser therapy has been used to treat port-wine stains, experience is limited with lymphangioma circumscriptum. CO_2 laser has been used more extensively.

Although the CO_2 laser and pulse-dye laser have been used to treat lymphangioma circumscriptum, wide surgical excision has been the standard of care for localized lesions. More extensive lesions that would require development of large flaps would best be managed with an initial attempt at laser ablation. Recurrence would be a strong possibility. The same may be said for wide local excision. It is possible for the lesion to return if the deeper communicating lymph channels persist and result in surface eruption of recurrent vesicles. Frozen section to clear margins (lateral and deep) may assist in surgical excision of lymphangioma circumscriptum.

Progressive Therapeutic Options

1. Reassurance if symptoms are not significant.
2. For well-localized lesions, wide local excision with an effort to remove the deep communicating channels (may assess margins by frozen section).
3. Laser ablation of lesions using the CO_2 laser.
4. For lesions with a significant red blood cell component, pulse-dye laser therapy may be considered.

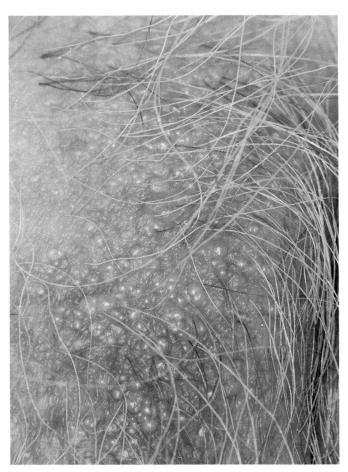

Figure 10.2. Multiple labial vesicles in patient with a history of prior radiotherapy for endometrial carcinoma.

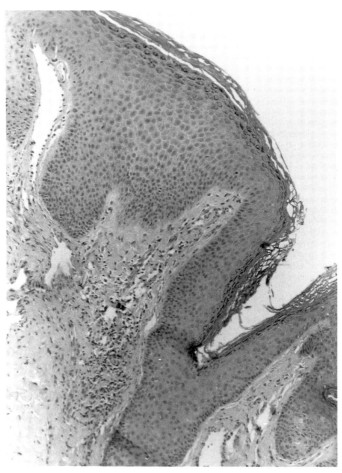

Figure 10.3. Lymphangioma circumscriptum. Vascular spaces are evident immediately beneath the epithelium. These spaces contain acellular eosinophilic fluid. The surface epithelium is elevated above the vesicle and is somewhat thinned.

11

PEDIATRICS

Adhesion/Agglutination

DEFINITION

Fusion of the labia minora results in labial adhesion or agglutination.

GENERAL FEATURES

The incidence of childhood labial agglutination is unknown, although it appears to be a rare problem. The etiology of the condition is poorly understood. Labial agglutination may be a consequence of a developmental abnormality (congenital) or may evolve as a consequence of labial and vestibular irritation initiating denuded epithelial surfaces that adhere to one another as a consequence of their close proximity.

CLINICAL PRESENTATION

The usual patient with labial adhesions will be brought to the clinic by her concerned mother who has noted no orifice at the vaginal opening. She will describe what appears to be an abnormality and will request further evaluation. Occasionally a child with labial adhesion will present with recurrent vaginal infections and urinary difficulties such as cystitis. The latter will be the case especially if labial fusion has resulted in almost complete obliteration of the vestibule.

MICROSCOPIC FEATURES

This clinical finding does not require biopsy. The vestibular epithelium of the child, with the exception of the newborn, is not glycogen rich and is nonkeratinized. No specific pathologic findings are known to be associated with labial agglutination of the newborn. In some societies, where female circumcision is practiced, labial agglutination is relatively common and may be associated with introital stenosis and keratinous cysts.

ADJUNCTIVE STUDIES

None.

DIFFERENTIAL DIAGNOSIS

The patient with a markedly adherent introitus may create concerns that one is dealing with an atretic vaginal canal of mullerian agenesis or androgen insensitivity syndrome. Placement of a lubricated cotton swab within the introital orifice will demonstrate the thin groove representing the adherent labia.

CLINICAL BEHAVIOR AND TREATMENT

For the asymptomatic child with labial agglutination that is too adherent to separate gently in the office, topical estrogen cream, applied once per evening for 2 weeks may resolve the agglutination and typically no further therapy is warranted. It is not in the patient's best interest to undergo general anesthesia for separation of the labia unless symptoms warrant such an invasive procedure. If the patient suffers from recurrent vaginal infections or bladder infections, then the procedure is indicated. If indications are present for the procedure, and gentle traction in the office demonstrates markedly agglutinated labia, then the procedure is best accomplished under appropriate anesthesia. Usually, placement of a probe or cotton swab to the adhesion, with gentle traction toward the perineum, will result in separation of the labia. Without postoperative separation of these denuded epithelial surfaces, fusion will recur. A time-honored approach to this problem has been the daily application of estrogen cream to the introitus. Although no pharmacologic data exist to support the antiadhesion benefit of estrogen creams, the effect may be related to maturation of the epithelium of the labia minora and vestibule. Topical estrogen is regularly used and is often successful. It may be that the benefit of the application is in part mechanical and that daily separation of the labia while applying the estrogen cream allows for epithelialization to occur and diminishes the chance of subsequent adhesion of the labia. This approach may be used as a substitute for surgery in the patient who has evidence of minimal agglutination.

Parents of the infant should be reassured that there is no evidence of a major abnormality, and if the infant is asymptomatic, the parents may be reassured that the labial orifice may expand on its own with the passage of time.

Progressive Therapeutic Options

1. In the asymptomatic patient observation alone with reassurance should be adequate. If the parent wishes "to intervene," daily application of estrogen cream for 2 weeks may be attempted, accompanied by gentle traction.

2. For the symptomatic patient, attempt *gentle* separation in the office. Markedly adherent labia will require lysis in the operating room if there is no response to topical estrogen. A "pediatric pain cocktail" may be administered to avoid anesthesia; however, close cardiopulmonary monitoring will be necessary. Postoperative daily separation of the labia by the parent is mandatory until reepithelialization has been completed. Estrogen cream may be applied during these daily efforts.

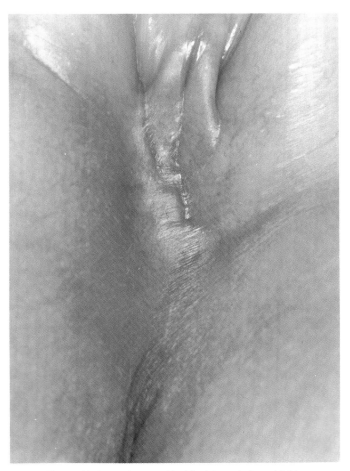

Figure 11.1. A 2-year-old girl with agglutinated labia.

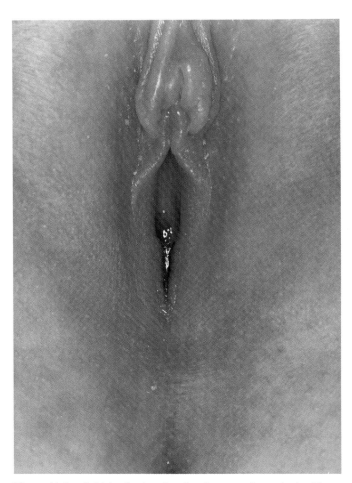

Figure 11.2. Labial adhesions lysed under general anesthesia. The patient's family was advised to maintain separation. One year later agglutination had recurred and the patient was followed without further intervention.

Condylomata Acuminata, Childhood

DEFINITION

Condylomata acuminata is derived from the Greek phrase for caruncle and the Latin phrase for sharply pointed and as such the terminology adequately defines the condition caused by human papillomavirus.

GENERAL FEATURES

Human papillomavirus appears to be responsible for the most common sexually transmitted disease seen by obstetricians and gynecologists in the 1990s. Increasingly, sexually active adolescents present with obvious venereal warts (or less obvious abnormal cervical cytology) as a consequence of human papillomavirus infection. These vulvar venereal warts also may be observed in early infancy and may be acquired during transmission through an infected birth canal or as a consequence of sexual abuse. The incubation period for human papillomavirus may be prolonged, and clinical evidence of a viral infection acquired during transmission through an infected birth canal may not be apparent for months or perhaps years after birth. Often in children the actual mode of transmission remains unknown. With the advent of sexual activity in early to late adolescence the mode of transmission becomes much more apparent.

CLINICAL PRESENTATION

The child with vulvar condylomata usually will be brought to the physician for evaluation of the warty lesions. Often this may be delayed and the process may be diffuse when first seen by the physician. Immunosuppressed patients, especially children with diabetes, may manifest diffuse disease. In such patients it is not uncommon to see warts elsewhere on the body surface.

MICROSCOPIC FEATURES

See condylomata acuminatum, Chapter 9.

ADJUNCTIVE STUDIES

The child with condylomata acuminata should be suspect for other venereal diseases and appropriate studies should be obtained. These would include cultures for gonorrhea, assays for chlamydia, serology for syphilis, and serology for human immunodeficiency virus. Consideration should also be given to evaluating for systemic diseases that may impair host immune defense, such as diabetes.

Consideration should also be given to the possibility of sexual abuse and inclusion of appropriate advocacy health care professionals and paraprofessionals should be initiated.

DIFFERENTIAL DIAGNOSIS

Those conditions that are seen in adults and may be confused with condylomata acuminata are much less frequent in children. Still, one must consider certain entities as potential diagnoses. Small papillary projections, often with centrally umbilicated centers, may be confused for condylomata acuminata; however, they are more likely to be lesions of molluscum contagiosum. When uncertainty exists, biopsy may be performed. Rarely molluscum contagiosum will present as large, fleshy tumors, and diagnosis will be impossible without histology. The large, broad-based lesions of secondary syphilis, condylomata lata, may be confused with condylomata acuminata and may have been treated inappropriately with topical desiccant agents. The clinician must remember that the child demonstrating evidence of one sexually transmitted disease must be considered at risk for other such disease. To differentiate condylomata acuminata from condylomata lata, one may rely upon dark-field or immunofluorescent examination of scrapings from the moist lata lesions, serology, and histology (as needed).

CLINICAL BEHAVIOR AND TREATMENT

The therapy for condylomata acuminata in childhood is much the same as that performed for adult patients. The reader is referred to the section on condylomata acuminata in the text. Immunosuppressed patients, such as diabetic patients, who require laser ablation of condylomata acuminata may benefit from augmentation with interferon injections into the vulvar skin; however, interferon-α has not been approved for use in children or patients under the age of 18. One must also remember that when dealing with young infants who have condylomata acuminata, blood loss associated with laser therapy must be monitored carefully. For the clinician who is accustomed to patients losing blood during vulvar ablations, the absolute amount of blood loss in a child will represent a greater proportion of actual blood volume than is seen in an adult. Appropriate hemostasis is mandatory, and volume repletion should be meticulous. Postoperative care will be dependent upon careful parental instruction concerning hygiene. Daily and frequent sitz baths may keep the lasered bed of vulvar skin clean and free of infection. It would behoove the clinician to see the treated child frequently to manage early infection before a significant infection evolves.

Progressive Therapeutic Options

1. For small lesions, use topical desiccants such as trichloroacetic or bichloroacetic acid or resin of podophyllin applied at weekly intervals. If multiple and frequent applications appear likely, then consideration should be given to one laser session.

2. For patients who wish to manage lesions at home, self-treatment or preferably parental treatment may be accomplished with podofilox solution applied twice daily for 3 days, followed by 4 days of abstinence, repeated for a total of 4 cycles. This should not be used in pregnant patients.

3. For patients with extensive disease, consider laser ablation. Large, bulky lesions may be more rapidly excised sharply or with electrical current. Therapy may then be augmented with the CO_2 laser at the same session.

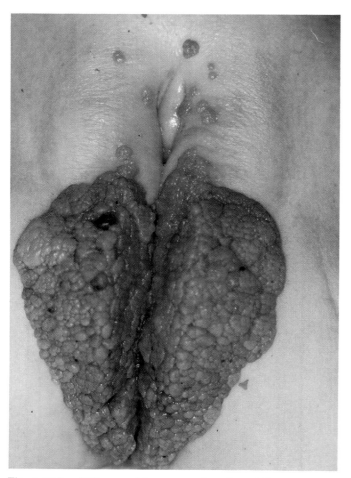

Figure 11.3. Diffuse condylomata acuminata in an infant.

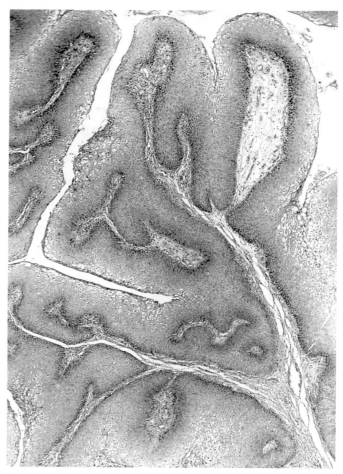

Figure 11.4. Condyloma acuminatum in a child. The papillomatous growth, with fibrovascular cords underlying the hyperplastic epithelium, is evident. The cellular features include koilocytoses and some lack of cellular maturation.

Hymen (Imperforate, Cribriform)

DEFINITION

An imperforate hymen results from failure of embryonic canalization of the endoderm of the urogenital sinus, resulting in a lack of communication between the vagina and the vestibule. Partial canalization results in a hymen with one or more small orifices (cribriform hymen).

GENERAL FEATURES

This condition is uncommon and is rarely diagnosed before menarche, at which point outflow obstruction becomes symptomatic.

CLINICAL PRESENTATION

The typical patient with an imperforate hymen will present at the age of menarche complaining of severe lower abdominal discomfort. This discomfort may have been noted cyclically for 1–3 months or longer. Upon questioning concerning menstruation, the patient will have noted no menstrual effluent. Examination may be difficult secondary to the significant degree of discomfort experienced by the patient. Abdominal examination may demonstrate a mass in the lower abdomen that represents an hematocolpos. Introital examination will demonstrate a distended hymen and no orifice opening into the vestibule other than the urethral meatus. Rectal examination will demonstrate a mass in the lower abdomen that will usually be quite tender.

Occasionally a patient with a partially canalized hymen will be seen in the premenarchal years with complaints of recurrent vaginal infection. On examination, a small opening or openings may be noted and the term cribriform hymen is applied to this situation.

ADJUNCTIVE STUDIES

The patient with an imperforate hymen may be evaluated with an ultrasound to define the hematocolpos and confirm the etiology of the pelvic mass.

DIFFERENTIAL DIAGNOSIS

In the newborn infant with a lower abdominal mass, the possibility of an imperforate hymen may be a consideration; however, careful examination of the introitus may demonstrate an opening that will prove to be urethra when followed endoscopically into the bladder. If an antecedent ultrasound has demonstrated a cystic structure in the lower abdomen, the possibility of hydrometrocolpos secondary to a transverse vaginal septum related to the McKusick-Kaufman syndrome should be considered. This condition also may be diagnosed antepartum on a screening ultrasound that demonstrates hydronephrosis and a cystic pelvic mass. This syndrome is secondary to incomplete fusion of the Mullerian tubes and the urogenital sinus, and not secondary to failure of canalization of the hymen.

MICROSCOPIC FEATURES

Resected tissue from the imperforate hymen has stratified squamous epithelium that is not keratinized present on both the vaginal and vulvar surface. It can be distinguished readily from tissue resected from transverse vaginal septum, which has stratified squamous epithelium on the vulvar surface and columnar epithelium, usually of endocervical type, on the vaginal surface.

CLINICAL BEHAVIOR AND TREATMENT

An imperforate hymen should be incised in the operating room under appropriate anesthesia. The recommended approach is placement of cruciate incisions in the distended hymen. The resultant triangular segments of hymen may be excised at or near their bases, and vaginal epithelium may then be sutured to vestibular epithelium with interrupted absorbable sutures. There is no need to perform invasive procedures in the vagina or the uterus at the time of this drainage. Drainage is easily accomplished and uterine curettage is not indicated to drain the concurrent hematometra. A patient with symptomatic cribriform hymen should also undergo excision of the hymen under appropriate anesthesia.

Progressive Therapeutic Option

1. Incision and excision of the hymen.

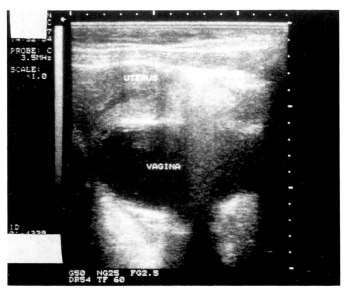

Figure 11.5. Ultrasound of hematocolpos secondary to imperforate hymen.

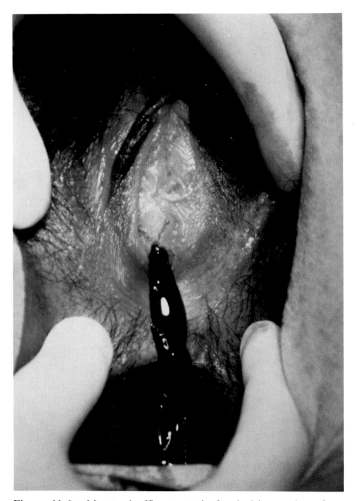

Figure 11.6. Menstrual effluent noted after incising an imperforate hymen.

Lentigo Simplex and Vulvar Melanosis

DEFINITION

Lentigo simplex is a hyperpigmented macular lesion resulting from excess production of melanin by melanocytes.

GENERAL FEATURES

This condition is more commonly seen in adults but on rare occasion may be seen in infants, and is often confused with a nevus.

CLINICAL PRESENTATION

Lesions will be asymptomatic and the usual cause for presentation is parental concern about the hyperpigmented lesion discovered on examination of the child. The lesion will be macular and dark. There will be no variegated appearance of the overlying epithelium. Coloring will be uniform.

MICROSCOPIC FEATURES

Lentigo simplex is clinically a pigmented lesion 4 mm or less in diameter. The keratinocytes in and near the basal layer and sometimes in the upper epidermis contain cytoplasmic melanin granules. Functional melanocytes are also present. The epithelium may be relatively similar to the adjacent epithelium, but may be acanthotic, with clubbed rete. A slight chronic inflammatory infiltrate may be seen beneath the pigmented lesion.

Vulvar melanosis is characterized by pigmented areas on the labia minora and/or majora, which may be single or multiple. The pigmented areas typically exceed 4 mm in diameter. Melanosis has histologic findings essentially the same as lentigo simplex; however, acanthosis and inflammation typically are not seen.

ADJUNCTIVE STUDIES

None.

DIFFERENTIAL DIAGNOSIS

Of primary concern is that the patient may have a nevus or dysplastic nevus and that with the passage of time a melanoma may evolve. Histologic evaluation is necessary for final diagnosis.

CLINICAL BEHAVIOR AND TREATMENT

Hyperpigmented nevi in childhood may have an increased risk of malignant degeneration during the life of the patient, and strong consideration should be given to removing them. This is especially true of the vulva, where examination is often difficult. Lentigo simplex cannot be differentiated clinically from a nevus, and histology is necessary for final disposition. Excisional biopsy is warranted.

Progressive Therapeutic Option

1. Excisional biopsy.

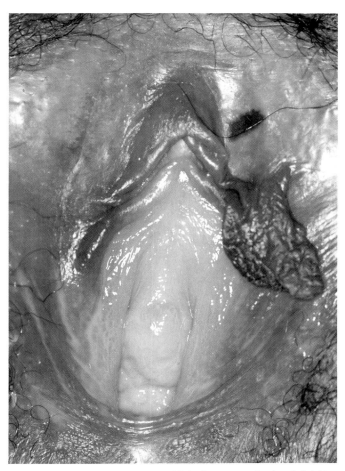

Figure 11.7. A 14-year-old girl with bothersome redundant left labium minus. At patient's and family's request, the labium was reduced surgically. In addition, the hyperpigmented left vulvar lesion was removed and found to be histologically consistent with melanosis.

Lichen Sclerosus

DEFINITION

Lichen sclerosus is a chronic dermatologic condition associated with epithelial thinning, inflammation, shrinkage, and agglutination of the labia.

GENERAL FEATURES

Lichen sclerosus is most commonly seen in perimenopausal and postmenopausal women. Rarely is it seen in the pediatric population. The etiology is unknown, although various mechanisms have been proposed, including immunology, genetics, and androgen receptor inactivity or deficiency.

CLINICAL PRESENTATION

Pediatric patients exhibiting changes of lichen sclerosus may be brought to the clinician for examination by a concerned mother who has noted the obvious epithelial thinning or lichenification. The symptomatic patient usually will complain of pruritus. On examination, the parchmentlike epithelium will be observed. In early stages, this will be a macular-appearing epithelium, but as irritation and self-induced trauma from scratching increase, the disease may be more plaquelike. The diagnosis is usually based on visual inspection. Biopsy in this age group is traumatic, but may be considered if marked uncertainty exists concerning the diagnosis.

MICROSCOPIC FINDINGS

Distinctive features of lichen sclerosus include loss of rete ridges, an edematous appearance of the dermis immediately beneath the epithelium, with a homogenization of the dermis, and apparent decrease of dermal vessels. Immediately beneath this dermal change, lymphocytes are present that are primarily localized between the junction of the edematous and normal-appearing deeper dermis. Depending on the duration of the process, its location, and external trauma secondary to scratching, the morphologic features can be highly variable. In very early lichen sclerosus, the subepithelial edematous area may be only focal, and rete ridges may still be relatively intact. Few inflammatory cells may be identified in the deeper dermis. In some cases, subepithelial bullae may be evident. Melanosomes and melanocytes typically are absent. If pruritis and excoriation have occurred, erosion or ulceration may be also present and are associated with focal acute and chronic inflammation. Blood may be found immediately beneath the epithelium and in the superficial dermis, due to localized subepidermal bleeding. In advanced cases, the epithelium may vary from very thinned to markedly thickened and hyperkeratotic. The dermal changes become more pronouced and the thickness of the involved dermis may increase and be more sclerotic. In the late stages, it may be impossible definitively to distinguish lichen sclerosus from advanced lichen planus. Morphae (localized scleroderma) also may be difficult to exclude. Topical corticosteroid therapy can improve the microscopic features of lichen sclerosus; however, pathologic findings may persist far after the clinical symptoms and general clinical appearance have improved. A similar situation may be observed in children with genital lichen sclerosus, where, with the onset of puberty, the symptoms and physical findings of lichen sclerosus may improve or regress. Biopsy will identify persistent disease if specifically sought.

DIFFERENTIAL DIAGNOSIS

Vitiligo may also present as white epithelium on the vulva. This condition is rarely symptomatic. It is symmetric and macular. If the vulvar skin has been irritated and is ecchymotic, then vulvovaginal candidiasis must be considered and an appropriate KOH preparation obtained.

CLINICAL BEHAVIOR AND TREATMENT

The disease will often undergo remission at the onset of adrenarche and menarche. This observation has supported the contention that androgen insensitivity or absence may be a prelude to the development to the condition. Although topical testosterone application has been used in adults to manage lichen sclerosus, current therapy for lichen sclerosus employs topical corticosteroids, usually medium to high-potency steroids daily until response occurs, then tapering frequency to maintain control of the process. The masculinizing effects of testosterone on children are unacceptable. An alternative approach is topical application of progesterone in oil (400 mg may be mixed with 4 oz of aquaphor and applied twice daily).

Progressive Therapeutic Options

1. Reassurance that often the condition will regress as the child progresses through adrenarche and menarche.
2. Progesterone in oil (400 mg in 4 oz of aquaphor) applied twice daily.

3. Betamethasone valerate 0.1% ointment (Valisone) applied once or twice daily for 1–2 weeks, or until symptoms regress, then taper frequency.

4. High-potency topical corticosteroids (Temovate, 0.05% cream) twice per day for 2–3 weeks, then taper to twice per week or less often to minimize use.

Redundant Labium Minus

DEFINITION

Elongation of a labium minus is referred to clinically as a redundant labium minus.

GENERAL FEATURES

Excessive elongation of a labium minus or both labia majora is rarely seen and more rarely is it symptomatic.

CLINICAL PRESENTATION

The symptomatic patient will complain of a sense of discomfort and perhaps irritation associated with the elongated tissue, especially noted when walking or when having intercourse.

MICROSCOPIC FEATURES

It is an unusual situation when the labia minora need to be resected due to hypertrophy. When resected the labia minora may have hyperkeratotic areas, interstitial edema, and fibrosis. The labia minora do not contain glandular elements or sebaceous glands. When sebaceous glands are seen in such resected specimens, they represent more peripheral tissues excised from near the base of the labia minora.

ADJUNCTIVE STUDIES

None.

DIFFERENTIAL DIAGNOSIS

No other entities are to be considered.

CLINICAL BEHAVIOR AND TREATMENT

The symptomatic adult redundant labium minus may be removed easily in the clinic with appropriate local anesthesia. The infant or child with such a condition may not be a candidate for local anesthesia and removal and may require an excision in the operating room. The excess tissue is removed and the skin is then approximated with interrupted absorbable suture material. The patient with no symptoms but concerns about the excess tissue may be assured that this is a normal variant and no therapy is indicated.

Progressive Therapeutic Options

1. Reassurance.
2. If symptomatic, excision and approximation of skin with interrupted absorbable suture material.

12

TRAUMA

Adhesions

DEFINITION

Adhesions are bands of fibrous tissue that occur as a consequence of normal wound physiology when denuded areas of epithelium are apposed.

GENERAL FEATURES

Vulvar adhesions are rare in the adult population. They are most commonly noted to occur after a vaginal birth when vulvar lacerations are followed by apposition of denuded tissue planes. They may be seen in neonates as labial adhesions associated with inflammatory dermatoses, and related to female circumcision.

CLINICAL PRESENTATION

The adult patient with vulvar adhesions may present with discomfort noted at the introitus. If the adhesions are strategically located and obstruct the normal urinary stream, then spraying may be noted with micturition. Intercourse may be painful. Bands of fibrous tissue may be noted across the introitus.

MICROSCOPIC FINDINGS

Excised adhesions have microscopic features of scar with thinning of the epithelium and fibrosis of the underlying dermis with localized loss of skin appendages. Chronic inflammation may be present with recent or irritated adhesions.

ADJUNCTIVE STUDIES

No adjunctive studies are needed to evaluate the patient with vulvar adhesions, believed to be secondary to trauma of childbirth.

DIFFERENTIAL DIAGNOSIS

The diagnosis of vulvar adhesions secondary to trauma is self-evident. This condition is not to be confused with a partially perforate hymen because the bands are distal to the hymen and are primarily vestibular in location.

CLINICAL BEHAVIOR AND TREATMENT

Symptomatic adhesions may be lysed easily in the clinic. A small wheal of topical anesthetic may be injected at the base of each origin or insertion before incising and excising the adhesion. To prevent reformation it will be necessary for the patient to keep the tissue planes distinct from one another, not allowing apposition of the medial edges of the vestibule or labia minora. Although estrogen creams traditionally have been applied to the vulva and vestibule to prevent reformation of adhesions after lysis, there is no evidence to support a pharmacologic role of the estrogen in preventing adhesions. The more likely mode of action is that daily application of the cream mechanically prevents apposition of tissue planes and allows healing to occur.

Progressive Therapeutic Option

1. In the symptomatic patient, after appropriate topical anesthesia, the adhesions may be excised easily in the clinic. Excision should be followed

by daily efforts on the part of the patient to keep the labia separated for varying periods of time to allow local healing without adherence of the labia or vestibule to the contralateral side. Estro-gen creams may be applied topically to assist the patient in massaging the area to prevent apposition, although no pharmacologic role of the estrogen creams has been demonstrated.

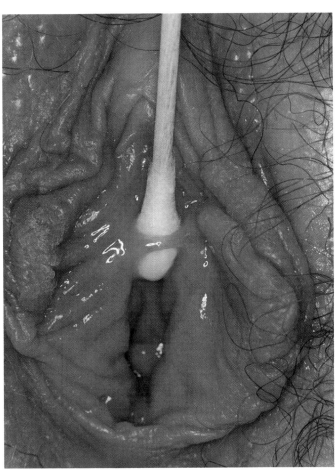

Figure 12.1. Painful adhesion noted after obstetric laceration. Adhesion was excised in the clinic.

Anoperineal Fistula

DEFINITION

An anoperineal fistula is a communication between the anus and the perineal body.

GENERAL FEATURES

A fistula involving the perineum or vestibule and communicating with the anus or rectum is almost invariably a consequence of a postobstetric event. Vaginal delivery may result in laceration of the anal sphincter and anal and rectal mucosa. Although this is repaired, dehiscence of the repair will result in a fistula tract.

CLINICAL PRESENTATION

The patient will present complaining of feculant material passing through the perineum or vestibule. If the anal sphincter has been disrupted, then fecal incontinence may be a significant symptom.

ADJUNCTIVE STUDIES

Evaluation of the rectal and anal mucosa for evidence of inflammatory bowel disease should be accomplished. Symptoms or findings suggestive of inflammatory bowel disease would warrant radiographic and endoscopic evaluation of the gastrointestinal tract.

DIFFERENTIAL DIAGNOSIS

As noted, the differential diagnosis would include inflammatory bowel disease, which should be suspected in patients with appropriate symptoms or findings (friable anal and rectal mucosa). The appearance of a fistula in a patient who has not experienced a vaginal delivery should raise the suspicion of inflammatory bowel disease, lymphogranuloma venereum, and carcinoma. Fistulae observed with lymphogranuloma venereum are often multiple and are associated with edema of the external genitalia, resulting in the anogenital syndrome. Appropriate serologic studies for the precipitating chlamydial organisms should be obtained. If carcinoma is suspected, then appropriate biopsies should be obtained.

MICROSCOPIC FEATURES

Fistulous tracts that communicate from the anal or bowel mucosa to the vulvar skin, vestibule, or vagina are often lined, in part, by squamous epithelium from the exterior epithelium. A marked acute and chronic inflammatory infiltrate is present in the tissue immediately adjacent to the fistula. In some cases, foreign body giant cells and polarizable foreign material may be found in the tract. On occasion, suture material or other foreign material may be within, or embedded in the wall, of the tract.

CLINICAL BEHAVIOR AND TREATMENT

Rarely a minute fistula resulting from obstetric trauma may heal spontaneously. Usually, surgical repair will be necessary. This repair should be accomplished as soon as the incision is free of evidence of infection. Often the anal sphincter will be involved in the fistulous tract and it will be necessary to reapproximate the anal sphincter as well as the rectal walls. The fistula tract may be defined with a lacrimal probe or may be delineated with methylene blue injected into the tract before incision. The excision and repair should be accomplished in the operating room under appropriate anesthesia. A preoperative bowel preparation with GoLYTELY or with colonic enemas should be accomplished. Broad-spectrum antibiotics should be administered before surgery to decrease colony counts within the surgical incision. The tract should be excised and the rectal wall should be approximated with interrupted 3–0 polyglactin 910 or similar absorbable suture. A reinforcing second layer of 2–0 polyglactin 910 should be placed securely in the muscularis of the bowel wall in an interrupted fashion. The anal sphincter may be approximated with three or four interrupted stitches of 0 absorbable suture material that include the muscle and capsule in the repair. With cephalic extension of the fistula, consideration should be given to approximating the levator ani muscles to reinforce the surgical repair and to augment the perineum. Perineal and vestibular skin may be approximated with running subcuticular 3–0 absorbable suture material. Postoperatively the patient may be managed as an outpatient with 7–10 days of an elemental diet, stool softeners, and sitz baths. The patient may benefit in the first 24 hours from an ice pack. Pain is usually controlled with oral analgesics.

Progressive Therapeutic Option

1. Excision and multilayer closure under broad-spectrum prophylactic antibiotics after appropriate bowel preparation with GoLYTELY or high colonic enemas.

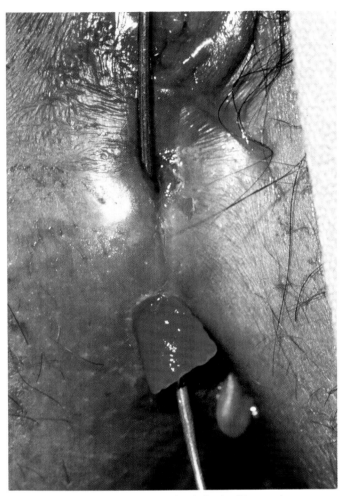

Figure 12.2. Postobstetric anoperineal fistula. Note exuberant granulation tissue. Sound demonstrates fistula tract. Tract was excised and closed primarily without recurrence.

Bullet Wound

DEFINITION

A bullet wound is a consequence of penetration of vulvar tissue planes by a metal projectile delivered by an explosive charge.

GENERAL FEATURES

With the increasing prevalence of weapons in the population and accelerating levels of violence, bullet injuries to the female genitalia may be expected to increase in frequency.

CLINICAL PRESENTATION

Depending upon the caliber of the weapon used and the trajectory of the projectile, vulvar findings may be minimal or massive. A small-caliber, hand-held weapon fired tangentially into the lower abdomen may result in a trajectory that terminates in the vulva, with minimal vulvar damage. Conversely, a large-gauge, pellet-containing weapon applied to the vulva before discharge will create massive, life-threatening injury.

ADJUNCTIVE STUDIES

Depending upon the entry site and the severity of damage, endoscopic studies of the bladder, urethra, bowel, and direct visualization of the peritoneal cavity to rule out visceral damage may be necessary.

MICROSCOPIC FEATURES

There is a considerable body of forensic pathology literature describing and defining entry and exit bullet wounds, and the distinction is often of critical importance in criminal investigations. Entry wounds, if occurring in close proximity to the weapon, usually will show evidence of gun powder and bullet or clothing fragments embedded about the entry site. Small tears, running parallel to the axis of the wound, may be evident. The entry site often appears to have relatively smooth margins appearing as a punched-out hole.

A bullet exit site may be highly variable, depending upon the velocity and type of the bullet and whether or not the skin of the exit site was supported (i.e., against a fixed surface) or free. In general, the higher the velocity of the bullet, the larger and more disrupted the exit site. The edges of the wound may appear serrated and torn, giving the wound a stellate appearance.

CLINICAL BEHAVIOR AND TREATMENT

Initial therapy will be designed to stabilize the patient and evaluate for vital structure trauma associated with the vulvar wound. In the absence of vascular instability or other organ trauma, the local vulvar wound should be treated surgically as indicated. Massive injuries may require debridement and delayed closure or healing by secondary intention. Ultimately, vaginal and vulva reconstruction may be necessary. If the projectile is contained within the vulvar tissues, then removal is indicated. Antibiotic prophylaxis may be warranted and the patient's tetanus immunizations should be updated.

Progressive Therapeutic Option

1. Local wound care should be accomplished and should consist of debridement and removal of the projectile with subsequent repair of the tissues as deemed appropriate by the level of injury and the presence of potentially infectious debris.

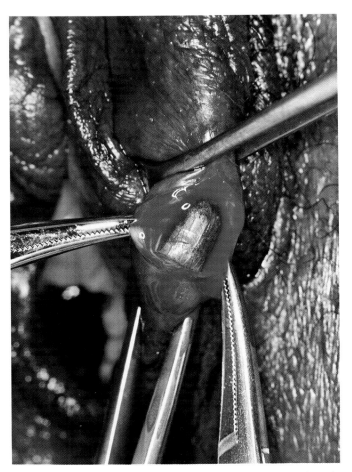

Figure 12.3. .22-caliber projectile lodged in left labium majus after entering suprapubic region and transversing space of Retzius without injuring bladder or urethra.

Granulation Tissue

DEFINITION

Granulation tissue is the term used to describe the granular-appearing surface of injured skin and subcutaneous tissues, which is characterized by neo-vascularization and epithelial migration, resulting in reepithelialization.

GENERAL FEATURES

The development of a granular-appearing epithelium in wounds allowed to heal by secondary intention is a normal process. Depending upon the size of the wound, this process, which results in a re-epithelialized surface, may take weeks to months. Within the lower reproductive tract, the vagina, and vestibule, this process may result in exuberant tissue that is polypoid in nature. Specifically, this tissue may be noted in vaginal incisions or lacerations, especially after hysterectomy or, rarely, after an episiotomy.

CLINICAL PRESENTATION

A patient with granulation tissue in an episiotomy site usually will present within the first few months after delivery complaining of pain, bleeding, and a palpable mass at the introitus. On examination, proliferative tissue will be noted in the region of the prior incision. This tissue will bleed easily to the touch and will be painful when manipulated.

MICROSCOPIC FEATURES

Granulation tissue typically is found where the epithelium surface is ulcerated. The granulation tissue is composed of prominent small, relatively thick-walled small vessels invested in a dermis that contains a mixture of acute and chronic inflammatory cells. The dermis may be highly variable in appearance, ranging from edematous to fibrotic. The epithelium adjacent to the ulcer with granulation tissue is usually relatively flattened and thin but may be hyperplastic if the ulcer is old or irritated.

ADJUNCTIVE STUDIES

When dealing with granulation tissue in an episiotomy site, no adjunctive studies are necessary unless there is suspicion that a rectovaginal fistula is present. In such an instance the patient will complain of feculent material in the vagina. The hypertrophied tissues will surround a small ostium, and passage of a lacrimal probe will demonstrate communication with the bowel lumen.

DIFFERENTIAL DIAGNOSIS

The presentation and findings are classic for this diagnosis. As noted in the adjunctive study section, it is important to rule out a fistula.

CLINICAL BEHAVIOR AND TREATMENT

This granulation tissue will be a persistent problem for the patient until it is removed. The base may be infiltrated with lidocaine and the process may be excised. The base may be chemically coagulated with silver nitrate. A small area of granulation tissue may be chemically coagulated with silver nitrate without excision. Topical cryotherapy or Monsel's solution are alternative therapies.

Progressive Therapeutic Options

1. Excision and chemical coagulation with silver nitrate.
2. Cryotherapy.
3. Topical Monsel's solution.

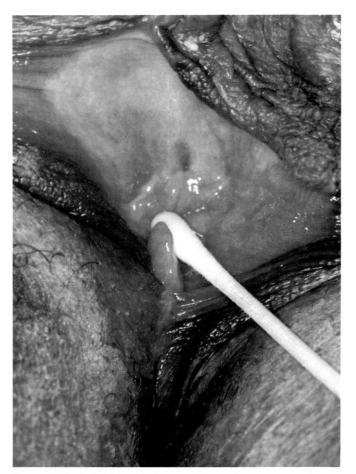

Figure 12.4. Painful granulation tissue in an episiotomy site. After local infiltration, the tissue was excised and the base was coagulated with silver nitrate.

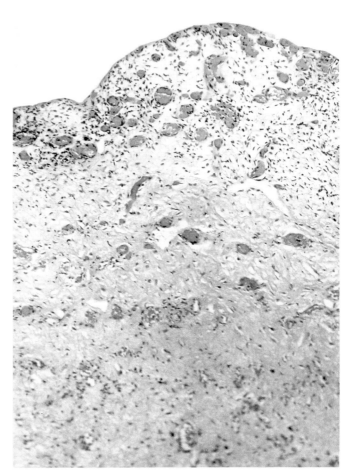

Figure 12.5. Granulation tissue. Multiple thin-walled small vessels are surrounded by an edematous fibrovascular tissue with mixed inflammatory cells. The surface is ulcerated.

Hematoma

DEFINITION

A hematoma is a collection of extravasated blood within the subcutaneous tissue of the vulva.

GENERAL FEATURES

Vulvar hematomas are relatively rare. They may occur as a consequence of obstetric trauma or as a consequence of blunt trauma to the vulva. Usually blunt trauma to the vulva is associated with a straddle injury and may be seen at any age. Such injuries may be noted in bicycle, gymnastic, and occupational accidents associated with loss of footing. Vulvar hematomas may also result from trauma associated with sexual assault. The vulva has a rich vascular supply derived primarily from branches of the internal pudendal artery, but secondarily derived anteriorly from branches of the external pudendal artery. This network of vessels, when forcefully compressed against the inferior fascia of the urogenital diaphragm, may rupture and extravasate. Usually this spread will be contained within the vulva between the planes of the inferior fascia of the urogenital diaphragm and the superficial perineal fascia (Colles' fascia), limited posteriorly by the aponeurosis of Colles' fascia with the superficial transverse perineal muscle and limited laterally by the aponeurosis of Colles' fascia with the ischiopubic ramus.

CLINICAL PRESENTATION

A patient with a vulvar hematoma will present with a stationary or expanding mass involving the vulva after experiencing blunt trauma to the region. The hematoma may be associated with ecchyomoses of the buttocks and thighs. The area will be quite tender. With significant trauma, concern should exist about the integrity of the anus, the urethral mechanism, and the bony structures of the pelvis (particularly the pubis and the symphysis pubis). Rarely will blood loss be so extensive as to result in hypovolemia; however, a young child experiencing such an injury may demonstrate a large hematoma, which, relative to the body's blood supply, would be sufficient to cause hypovolemia. Most vulvar hematomas are relatively small in size and often will be managed at home. Most hematomas evaluated by clinicians are relatively large in size, perhaps accounting for patients presenting for clinical management. A large hematoma may be associated with urinary retention secondary to mechanical obstruction or due to an associated urethral injury.

Rarely, a patient with a hematoma will not seek medical care and will present days later with an infected hematoma. The infection may derive from a laceration or puncture wound of the vulvar skin that has allowed ingress of bacteria.

The diagnosis of a vulva hematoma is usually obvious based upon clinical evaluation and the patient's immediate antecedent history. No biopsy is necessary.

MICROSCOPIC FINDINGS

Treatment of hematoma does not require biopsy or excision; however, hematomas may be incised and drained. An organized blood clot is usually found in resolving hematomas. The organized clot usually contains hemosiderin-laden macrophages. The age of the hematoma will influence the pathologic findings.

DIFFERENTIAL DIAGNOSIS

The differential diagnosis of a vulvar hematoma in the face of antecedent trauma is limited only to the diagnosis of vulvar hematoma. Rarely there will be no history of antecedent trauma, yet the clinical picture appears to be consistent with a hematoma. In such an instance, consideration should be given to a coagulopathy such as von Willebrand's disease, which may be associated with a spontaneous hematoma secondary to minimal trauma associated with routine daily activities. An expanding mass in the vulva without a history of trauma should also result in consideration of a Bartholin's cyst (or abscess), a lipoma, a hemangioma, or a canal of Nuck cyst.

CLINICAL BEHAVIOR AND TREATMENT

Most small vulvar hematomas require no intervention. Cold compresses traditionally have been used in the initial stages of formation. Pressure against the vulva, as against any area of bleeding within the body, will tamponade bleeding surfaces and allow the coagulation cascade to effect hemostasis. Expanding hematomas and large, symptomatic hematomas will require evacuation. They will require evacuation to control symptoms, particularly pain. There will be marked relief of the patient's discomfort with evacuation of an expanding or large hematoma. Evacuation and drainage of a vulvar hematoma will rarely result in isolation of any partic-

ular bleeding vessel. Usually the bleeding vessels
will have been tamponaded by the expanding hematoma or thrombose, and no specific bleeding site
will be identified. If generalized oozing is noted
within the cavity of the hematoma after evacuation,
then the space may be packed with an iodoform
gauze, which should be removed within 24 hours.
Generalized oozing also may be managed with
thrombin spray.

Urethral and anal injury should be excluded by
appropriate examination. A urinalysis may suffice
to rule out hematuria. Urinary retention will require
catheterization. Suspicion of urethral injury should
prompt urethroscopy/cystoscopy. Anal trauma generally can be excluded through digital examination.

An infected vulvar hematoma will require drainage and broad-spectrum antibiotic coverage.

Progressive Therapeutic Options

1. For a small relatively asymptomatic hematoma,
   cold compresses and observation.
2. For a symptomatic hematoma associated with
   urinary retention or hematuria, perform urethroscopy and cystoscopy to rule out urethral and
   bladder injury. Foley catheter urinary drainage
   may be necessary if pain precludes micturition.
3. For a symptomatic large hematoma or an expanding symptomatic hematoma, incise and
   drain the hematoma. If generalized oozing is visualized in the cavity of the hematoma, place a
   iodoform gauze packing, to be removed in 24
   hours.

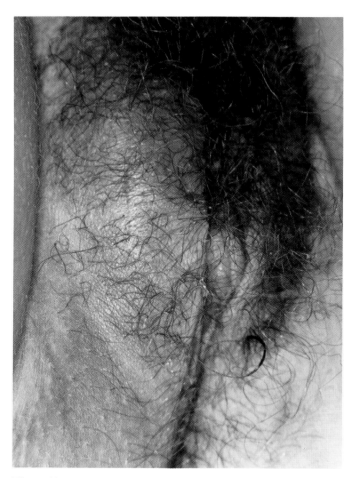

Figure 12.6. Right labial hematoma occurring after straddle injury. Ex-
pansion to 10 cm and inability to urinate prompted cystourethroscopy
with confirmation of no injury to the urethra or bladder. The hematoma
was evacuated and the patient was discharged on postoperative day 1.

Insect Bites and Stings

DEFINITION

Insects may inflict deadly venoms for purposes of immobilizing prey and defending territory.

GENERAL FEATURES

A multitude of biting and stinging insects may inflict trauma on unwary or unprotected persons. Usually the consequences of such bites or stings are a minor nuisance. In some instances, life-threatening responses are observed. Within the order Hymenoptera there are several stinging insects of major clinical importance. The family Vespidae includes yellow jackets, hornets, and wasps. The family Apidae includes honey bees and the family Formicidae includes fire ants. All of these insects may inject venom that contains proteins that may be allergenic and toxic. Biting insects are found in the orders of Acari (ticks) and Araneae (spiders). Ticks are especially noteworthy for diseases such as Lyme disease and Rocky Mountain spotted fever. Within the order Araneae, the most feared biting genera are Loxosceles (brown recluse spider) and Latrodectus (black widow spider). These spiders are known for the potentially fatal venom that may be injected into the site of their bites.

CLINICAL PRESENTATION

Most vulvar insect bites are of unknown etiology. Unless the patient has trapped the offending insect or unless it is still attached to the skin (i.e., a tick), the clinician will be faced with evaluating traumatized and often erythematous skin with no knowledge of the offending insect. The patient frequently will complain of a bite or sting and subsequent symptoms.

The stinging insects inject a venom that contains proteins that may induce a significant allergenic response. Included within the venom may also be alkaloids such as piperidione (fire ant venom) that may be hemolytic and cytotoxic. The patient will complain of local discomfort and itching. Rarely systemic manifestations as a response to the protein moiety may be life threatening. Anaphylactic shock with bronchial spasm, laryngeal edema, and hypotension may result in death without prompt intervention.

Spider bites usually occur on the extremities and rarely are seen in the genital region. When seen in the genital region they are usually associated with use of outside toilets and are usually secondary to Latrodectus bites (black widow spiders). Latrodectus venom is a neurotoxin. Within an hour after the venom has been injected, muscle cramping will commence involving the abdominal muscles, thighs, shoulders, and back. Life-threatening hypertension may evolve rapidly. The venom injected by the Loxosceles spiders is primarily cytotoxic, resulting in formation of a indurated, painful skin lesion that over the course of 4–7 days evolves into a sloughing necrotic ulcer. Rarely, systemic symptoms may result from such a bite, resulting in hemolysis and disseminated intravascular coagulation.

ADJUNCTIVE STUDIES

No adjunctive studies are necessary for the routine insect bite or sting.

DIFFERENTIAL DIAGNOSIS

The differential diagnosis of an insect bite or sting without the offending insect present includes contact dermatitis and herpes.

MICROSCOPIC FEATURES

Insect bites are characteristically superficial and deep inflammatory infiltrates. The type of insect bite or sting usually cannot be determined from the histopathologic features, although mosquito bites typically evoke an acute inflammatory cell response, with a late allergic response characterized by lymphocytes and plasma cells with infrequent eosinophils. Stinging insects, including wasps and bees, initially may evoke necrosis but in the later phases a subacute to chronic lymphocytic response will be seen. The chronic lymphocytic response may be exuberant with lymphoid follicles. This is also true for tick bites. In some cases careful sectioning may identify the stinger tract and residual insect stinger or feeling parts. This is especially true for bee and tick stings, respectively.

The brown recluse spider bite results in a necrotic ulcer with secondary perivasculitis and vascular necrosis. The inflammatory infiltrate includes chronic inflammatory cells and eosinophils.

CLINICAL BEHAVIOR AND TREATMENT

The standard approach to managing the Hymenoptera stings is to apply ice to the region of the bite and control itching with an oral antihistamine. A topical paste of meat tenderizer may be of value if applied early. With mild systemic symptoms, subcutaneous epinephrine may be administered as 0.01 mg/kg 1 to 1000 solution, not to exceed 0.5 mg.

With marked swelling, prednisone may be administered at a dose of 1–2 mg/kg/day for 5 days orally. Significant systemic reactions will require aggressive cardiopulmonary resuscitation. Airway establishment and correction of bronchial spasm will be essential. Circulation support will require intravenous access and fluid resuscitation. If subcutaneous epinephrine is ineffective, intravenous epinephrine will be necessary. Intravenous antihistamines such as diphenhydramine will be necessary, and intravenous steroids will assist in blocking a late response.

Latrodectus bites require routine local wound care and administration of tetanus prophylaxis as deemed appropriate. Control of pain and muscle relaxation usually will require intravenous morphine or meperidine and intravenous benzodiazepines such as diazepam or lorazepam. After appropriate skin testing, black widow antivenin should be administered.

Loxosceles spider bites should be managed with analgesics. If itching is present, oral antihistamines may be administered. Dapsone may assist early healing of the ulcer, but it should not be administered in patients who are glucose-6-phosphate dehydrogenase deficient. If Dapsone is used, then careful monitoring of blood parameters should be performed initially at weekly intervals. Special attention should be paid to complete blood cell counts. As with many vulvar conditions, the bite and subsequent ulcer may be managed with Burow's soaks. Heat should not be applied to the region.

For those stings and bites of unknown etiology without evidence of significant local or systemic reaction, local wound care with cool soaks in Burow's solution or local application of ice packs is often soothing. Oral diphenhydramine (Benadryl) or hydroxyzine (Atarax) may be administered to control pruritus.

Progressive Therapeutic Options

1. For a mild reaction to a bite or sting, ice packs and cool soaks in Burow's solution. Control pruritus with diphenhydramine (Benadryl) at 25–50 mg orally every 6 hours or hydroxyzine (Atarax) at 10–100 mg orally every 4–8 hours.
2. For minimal systemic reaction to a Hymenoptera sting, inject 0.01 mg/kg 1 to 1,000 epinephrine, not to exceed 0.5 mg, subcutaneously. If necessary, repeat dose at 15–20-minute intervals. Administer diphenhydramine as 10–50 mg intramuscularly.
3. For Latrodectus (black widow spider) bites, administer intravenous diazepam 2–10 mg to desired effect and control pain with intravenous morphine or meperidine. After skin sensitivity testing, administer antivenin, one vial in 50–100 mL of normal saline administered slowly over 30 minutes.
4. For Loxosceles (brown recluse spider) bites, local wound care and consider Dapsone at 50–100 mg orally every day. Screen for glucose-6-phosphate dehydrogenase deficiency before initiating and follow complete blood cell counts, liver enzymes, and renal function. Hemolysis and disseminated intravascular coagulation should be managed appropriately. Control itching with diphenhydramine at 25–50 mg orally every 6–8 hours.

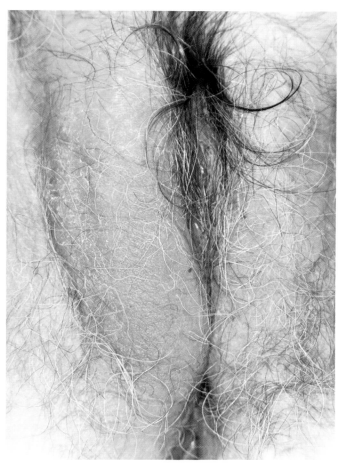

Figure 12.7. Right labial erythema and edema noted after an unknown (unidentified) insect bite/sting.

APPENDIX

Table A.1
Infectious Diseases of the Vulva

DISEASE	CAUSATIVE MICROORGANISM	SALIENT HISTOPATHOLOGIC FEATURES	DIAGNOSTIC METHODS
Condyloma acuminatum	Papillomavirus	Acanthosis, hyperkeratosis, parakeratosis, papillomatosis, perinuclear halo (koilocyte)	Histopathology Immunohistochemistry Molecular hybridization
Herpes genitalis	Herpes simplex hominis Type II	Intranuclear inclusions	Cytopathology, culture, serology
Syphilitic chancre	Treponema pallidum	Ulceration, chronic inflammation vasculitis	Dark-field, fluorescence, silver stain, serology
Condyloma lata	Treponema pallidum	Like chancre, with epithelial hyperplasia	Same as syphilitic chancre
Molluscum contagiosum	DNA poxvirus group	Intracytoplasmic inclusion	Cytopathology, histopathology
Granuloma inguinale	Calymmatobacterium granulomatis	Donovan bodies, granulomatous reaction without caseation, pseudoepitheliomatous hyperplasia	Giemsa stain, silver stain
Lymphogranuloma venereum	Chlamydia trachomatis	Granulomatous reaction without caseation	Serology
Tuberculosis	Mycobacterium tuberculosis	Acid-fast bacilli (AFB), granulomatous reaction with caseation	AFB stain, AFB culture
Chancroid	Haemophilus ducreyi	Granulomatous reaction without caseation	Culture, gram stain

From Wilkinson EJ. Benign diseases of the vulva. In: Kurman RJ, ed. Blaustein's Pathology of the Female Genital Tract. 4th ed. New York: Springer-Verlag, 1994.

Table A.2
Differential Diagnosis of Vesicular Bullous and Bullouslike Diseases of the Vulva

DISEASE	LOCATION OF VESICLE: SUBEPIDERMAL	INTRAEPIDERMAL AND/OR SUPRABASAL	ACANTHOLYSIS OF SUPRABASAL CELLS	SIGNIFICANT SYSTEMIC MANIFESTATION	IMMUNOFLUORESCENT LOCALIZATION
Pemphigus vulgaris	No	Yes	Yes	Yes	IgG intercellular
Pemphigus vegitans	No	Yes	Yes	No	IgG intercellular
Pemphigoid (bullous) (cicatricial pemphigoid)	Yes	No	No	Yes Localized scarring (sometimes debilitating)	IgG linear along basement membrane. IgA, IgM, C_3, C_5 may be in basement membrane
Herpes genitalis	Yes	No	No	Yes	C_3 linear along basement membrane. IgG may also be present. IgM, IgA are rare.
Polymorphic eruption of pregnancy, pruritic urticarial plaques and papules in pregnancy	Yes	No	No	Yes	Negative
Darier's disease	No	Yes	Yes, 3+ dyskeratosis	Yes	Negative
Warty dyskeratoma	No	Yes	Yes	No	Negative
Erythema multiforme (Stevens-Johnson syndrome)	No	Yes, necrotic keratinocytes, hydropic degeneration of basal keratinocytes	No	Yes	IgM Complement in and about superficial dermal vessels in some cases
Hailey-Hailey	No	Yes	Yes, 4+ No dyskeratosis	No	Negative
Localized acantholytic disease of the vulva	No	Yes	Yes	No	Negative
Benign chronic bullous disease of childhood (linear IgA disease)	Yes	No	Microabscesses in dermal papillae	No Flu-like symptoms may proceed findings	IgA linear along basement membrane. C_3, IgA, IgG, IgM may also be present.
Dermatitis herpetiformis	Yes	No	No	No Severe pruritus in some cases	IgA deposits in the tips of dermal papillae and/or along the basement membrane

From Wilkinson EJ. Benign diseases of the vulva. In: Kurman RJ, ed. Blaustein's Pathology of the Female Genital Tract, 4th ed. New York: Springer Verlag, 1994.

SELECTED READINGS

General

Abramowicz M. Drugs for sexually transmitted diseases. In: The Medical Letter on drugs and therapeutics. vol. 36, New Rochelle, NY; January 7, 1994.

Fitzpatrick TB, Eisen AZ, Wolff K, Freedberg IM, Austen KF. Dermatology in general medicine. 4th ed. New York: McGraw-Hill, 1993.

Friedrich EG Jr. In: Friedman EA, ed. Vulvar disease. 2nd ed. Philadelphia: WB Saunders, 1983.

Fu YS, Reagan JW. In: Bennington JL, ed. Pathology of the uterine cervix, vagina, and vulva, vol 21. Philadelphia: WB Saunders, 1989.

Habif TP. Clinical dermatology: a color guide to diagnosis and therapy. 2nd ed. St. Louis: CV Mosby, 1990.

Kaufman RH, Friedrich EG Jr, Gardner HL. Benign diseases of the vulva and vagina. 3rd ed. Chicago: Year Book, 1989.

Kurman RJ, Norris HJ, Wilkinson EJ. In: Rosai J, ed. Atlas of tumor pathology: tumors of the cervix, vagina, and vulva, vol. 4. Washington DC, Armed Forces Institute of Pathology, 1992.

Lever WF, Schaumburg-Lever G. Histopathology of the skin. 7th ed. Philadelphia: JB Lippincott, 1990.

McKee PH. In: Jowett M, Smillie, eds. Pathology of the skin with clinical correlations. Philadelphia: JB Lippincott, 1989.

Millikan LE. Drug eruptions (dermatitis medicamentosa). In: Moschella SL, Harley HJ, eds. Dermatology. 2nd ed. Philadelphia: WB Saunders; (1985):425–463.

Morse SA. Atlas of sexually transmitted diseases. Philadelphia: JB Lippincott, 1990.

O'Rahilly R, Muller F. Human embryology and teratology. New York: John Wiley & Sons, 1992.

Reed RJ. Neoplasms of the skin. In: Silverberg SG, ed. Principles and practice of surgical pathology. 2nd ed. New York: Churchill Livingstone, 1990:193–254.

Ridley CM. The vulva. New York: Churchill Livingstone, 1988.

Rook A, Dawber R. Diseases of the hair and scalp. 2nd ed. Boston: Blackwell Scientific Publications, 1991.

Rook AJ, Wilkinson DS, Ebling FJG. In: Champion RH, Burton JL, Ebling FJG, eds. Textbook of dermatology. 5th ed. Boston: Blackwell Scientific Publications, 1992.

Scully RE, Bonfiglio TA, Kurman RJ, Silverberg SG, Wilkinson EJ. WHO international histological classification of tumours. Histological typing of female genital tract tumours. 2nd ed. New York: Springer-Verlag, 1994.

Shelley WB, Shelley ED. Advanced dermatologic therapy. Philadelphia: WB Saunders, 1987.

Wilkinson EJ. Pathology of the vulva and vagina. vol. 9. New York: Churchill Livingstone, 1987.

Wilkinson EJ. Benign diseases of the vulva. In: Kurman RJ, ed. Blaustein's Pathology of the female genital tract. 4th ed. New York: Springer-Verlag, 1994:31–183.

Wilkinson EJ. Premalignant and malignant tumors of the vulva. In: Karman RJ, ed. Blaustein's pathology of the female genital tract. 4th ed. New York: Springer-Verlag, 1994:87–129.

Wilkinson EJ, Hardt NS. Vulva. In: Sternberg SS, ed. Histology for pathologists. New York: Raven Press, 1992;865–879.

Wisdom A. Color atlas of venereology. Chicago: Year Book, 1973.

Anatomy of the Vulva

Dickinson RL. Human sex anatomy. 2nd ed. Baltimore: Williams and Wilkins, 1949.

Edwards JNT, Morris HB. Langerhans cells and lymphocyte subset in the female genital tract. Br J Obstet Gynaecol 1985;92:974–982.

Fetissof F, Berger G, Dubois MP, Arbeille-Brassart B, Lansac J, Jm-Giao M, & Jopard P. Endocrine cells in the female genital tract. Histopathology 1985;9:133–145.

Freidrich EG, Jr. Vulvar disease. Philadelphia: WB Saunders, 1983.

Friedrich EG, Jr. Vulvar vestibulitis syndrome. J Reprod Med 1987;32:110–114.

Friedrich EG, Jr, Wilkinson EJ. Mucous cysts of the vulvar vestibule. Obstet Gynecol 1973;42:407–414.

Growdon WA, Fu Y, Lebberz TB, Rapkin A, Mason GD, Parks G. Pruritic vulvar squamous papillomatosis: evidence for human papillovavirus etiology. Obstet Gynecol 1985;66:564–568.

Hart DB: Selected papers in gynaecology and obstetrics. Edinburgh: W&AK Johnston, 1893.

Hu F. Melanocyte cytology in normal skin. In: Ackerman AB, ed. Masson Monographs in Dermatology-1. New York: Masson, 1981.

Kaufman RH, Friedrich EG, Gardner HL. Benign diseases of the vulva and vagina. 3rd ed. Chicago: Year-Book, 1989.

Krantz FK. Innvervation of the human vulva and vagina. Obstet Gynecol 1958;12:382–396.

Krantz KE. The anatomy and physiology of the vulva and vagina. In: Philipp EE, Barnes J, Newton M, eds. Scientific foundation of obstetrics and gynaecology, 2nd ed. London: Heinemann, 1977:65–78.

Lunde O. A study of body hair density and distribution in normal women. Am J Phys Anthropol 1984;64:179–184.

McKay M. Subsets of vulvodynia. J Reprod Med 1988;33:695–698.

Parmley T. Embryology of the female genital tract. In Kurman RJ, ed. Blaustein's pathology of the female genital tract. 3rd ed. New York: Springer Verlag, 1978:1–14.

Pyka R, Wilkinson EJ, Friedrich EG, Croker BP. The histology of vulvar vestibulitis syndrome. Int J Gynecol Oncol 1988;7:249–257.

Reid R, Greenberg MD, Daoud Y, Selvaggi S, Husain M, Wilkinson EJ. Colposcopic findings in women with vulvar pain syndromes: a preliminary report. J Reprod Med 1988;33:523–532.

Ridley CM. The vulva. New York: Churchill Livingstone, 1988:1–69.

Robboy SJ, Ross JS, Prat J, Keh PC, Welch WR. Urogenital sinus origin of mucinous and ciliated cysts of the vulva. Obstet Gynecol 1978;51:347–351.

Rorat E, Ferenczy A, Richart RM. Human Bartholin gland, duct, and duct cyst. Arch Pathol 1975;99:367–374.

Shatz P, Bergeron C, Wilkinson, EJ, Arseneau J, Ferenczy A. Vulvar intraepithelial neoplasia and skin appendage involvement. Obstet Gynecol 1989;74:769–774.

Wilkinson EJ. Pathology of the vagina. Curr Opin Obstet Gynecol 1991;3:553, 865–879.

Wilkinson EJ, Freidrich EG, Jr. Diseases of the vulva. In: Kurman RJ, ed. Blaustein's pathology of the female genital tract. 3rd ed. New York: Springer Verlag, 1987:36–96.

Wilkinson EJ, Hardt NS. Histology of the vulva. In Sternberg SS, ed. Histology for pathologists. New York: Raven Press; 1991:865–879.

Word B. Office treatment of cyst and abscess of Bartholin's gland duct. South Med J 1968;61:514–518.

Superficially Invasive Vulvar Carcinoma

Andersen BL, Hacker NF. Psychosexual adjustment after vulvar surgery. Obstet Gynecol 1983;62:457–462.

Berman ML, Soper JT, Creasman WT, Olt GW, DiSaia PJ. Conservative surgical management of superficially invasive stage I vulvar carcinoma. Gynecol Oncol 1989;35:352–357.

Boyce J, Fruchter RG, Kasambilides E, Nicastri AD, Sedlis A, Remy JC. Prognostic factors in carcinoma of the vulva. Gynecol Oncol 198520:364–377.

Buscema J, Stern JL, Woodruff JD. Early invasive carcinoma of the vulva. Am J Obstet Gynecol 1981;140:563–569.

Chafe W, Richards A, Morgan LS, Wilkinson EJ. Unrecognized invasive carcinoma in vulvar intraepithelial neoplasia (VIN). Gynecol Oncol 1988;31:154–165.

DiSaia PJ. Management of superficially invasive vulvar carcinoma. Clin Obstet Gynecol 1985;28:196–203.

Donaldson ES, Powell DE, Hanson MB, van Nagell JR. Prognostic parameters in invasive vulvar cancer. Gynecol Oncol 1981;11:184–190.

Dvoretsky P, Bonfiglio T, Helmkamp F, Ramsey G, Chuang C,

Beecham JB. The pathology of superficially invasive, thin vulvar squamous cell carcinoma. Int J Gynecol Pathol 1984;3:331–342.

FIGO News. Annual report on the results of treatment in gynecological cancer. Int J Gynaecol Obstet 1989;28:189–193.

Fu YS, Reagan JW, Townsend DE, et al. Nuclear DNA study of vulvar intraepithelial and invasive squamous neoplasms. Obstet Gynecol 1981;57:643–652.

Hacker NF, Berek JS, Lagasse LD, et al. Individualization of treatment for stage I squamous cell carcinoma of the vulva. Obstet Gynecol 1984;63(2):155–162.

Hacker NF, Vander Velden J. Conservative management of early vulvar cancer. Cancer 1993;71(Suppl):1673–1677.

Iversen T. New approaches to treatment of squamous cell carcinoma of the vulva. Clin Obstet Gynecol 1985;28:204–210.

Kelley JL III, Burke TW, Tornos C, et al. Minimally invasive vulvar carcinoma: an indication for conservative surgical therapy. Gynecol Oncol 1992;44:240–244.

Kneale BL. Microinvasive cancer of the vulva: report of the international society for the study of vulvar disease task force: Proceedings of the 7th World Congress of the ISSVD. J Reprod Med 1983;29:454–456.

Pickel H, Haas J. Microcarcinoma of the vulva. J Reprod Med 1986;31:831–835.

Rowley KC, Gallion HH, et al. Prognostic factors in early vulvar cancer. Gynecol Oncol 1988;31:43–49.

Schulz MJ, Penalver M. Recurrent vulvar carcinoma in the intervening tissue bridge in early invasive stage I disease treated by radical vulvectomy and bilateral groin dissection through separate incisions. Gynecol Oncol 1989;3:383–386.

Sedlis A, Homesley H, Bundy BN, et al. Positive groin lymph nodes in superficial squamous cell vulvar cancer. Am J Obstet Gynecol 1987;156:1159–1164.

Van der Velden J. Conservative management of early vulvar cancer. Cancer 1993;71(Suppl):1673–1677.

Wharton JT, Gallager S, Rutledge RN. Microinvasive carcinoma of the vulva. Am J Obstet Gynecol 1974;118:159–162.

Wilkinson EJ. Superficially invasive carcinoma of the vulva. In: Wilkinson EJ. ed. Contemporary issues in surgical pathology: pathology of the vulva and vagina. vol. 9. New York: Churchill Livingstone, 1987:103–117.

Wilkinson EJ. Superficially invasive carcinoma of the vulva. Clin Obstet Gynecol 1991;34:651–661.

Wilkinson EJ, Rico MJ, Pierson KK. Microinvasive carcinoma of the vulva. Int J Gynecol Pathol 1982;1:29–39.

Wilkinson EJ, Kneale B, Lynch PJ. International Society for the Study of Vulvar Disease: Report of the ISSVD Terminology Committee. J Reprod Med 1986;31:973–974.

Zaino RJ. Carcinoma of the vulva, urethra, and Bartholin's gland. In: Wilkinson EJ, ed. Contemporary issues in surgical pathology: pathology of the vulva and vagina. vol. 9. New York: Churchill Livingstone, 1987:119–154.

Zaino RJ, Husseinzadch N, Nahhas W, Mortel R. Epithelial alterations in proximity to invasive squamous carcinoma of the vulva. Int J Gynecol Pathol 1982;1:173–184.

REFERENCES

1. Addison WA, Livengood CH, Hill GB, Sutton GP, Fortier KJ. Necrotizing fasciitis of vulvar origin in diabetic patients. Obstet Gynecol 1984–5; 63:473.

2. Aneiros J, Belträn E, Garcia del Moral R, Nagoles FF Jr. Epithelioid leiomyoma of the vulva. Diagn Gynecol Obstet 1982; 4:351–356.

3. Avinoach I, Zirfkin HJ, Glezerman M. Proliferating trichilemmal tumor of the vulva. Case report and review of the literature. Int J Gynecol Pathol 1989; 8:163–168.

4. Axe S, Parmley T, Woodruff JD, Hlopak B. Adenomas in minor vestibular glands. Obstet Gynecol 1986; 68:16–18.

5. Balfour FJT, Vincenti AC. Idiopathic vulvar calcinosis. Histopathology 1991; 18:183–184.

6. Barnhill RL, Albert LS, Shama SK, Goldenhersh MA, Rhodes AR, Sober AJ. Genital lentiginosis: a clinical and histopathologic study. J Am Acad Dermatol 1990; 22:453–460.

7. Basta A, Madej JG Jr. Hidradenoma of the vulva. Incidence and clinical observations. Eur J Gynecol Oncol 1990; 11:185–189.

8. Bergeron C, Ferenczy A, Richart RM, Guralnick M. Micropapillomatosis labialis appears unrelated to human papillomavirus. Obstet Gynecol 1990; 76:281–286.

9. Berth-Jones J, Graham-Brown RA, Burns DA. Lichen sclerosus et atrophicus—a review of 15 cases in young girls. Clin Exp Dermatol 1991; 16:14–17.

10. Bonafe JL, Thibaut I, Hoff J. Introital adenosis associated with the Stevens-Johnson Syndrome. Clin Exp Dermatol 1990; 15:356–357.

11. Boyce DC, Valpey JM. Acute ulcerative vulvitis of obscure etiology. Obstet Gynecol 1971; 38:440.

12. Buchler DA, Sun F, Chaprevich T. A pilar tumor of the vulva. Gynecol Oncol 1978; 6:479–486.

13. Carli P, Cattaneo A, Pimpinelli N, Cozza A, Bracco G, Giannotti B. Immunohistochemical evidence of skin immune system involvement in vulvar lichen sclerosus et atrophicus. Dermatologica 1991; 182:18–22.

14. Carter J, Elliott P, Russell P. Bilateral fibroepithelial polypi of labium minus with atypical stromal cells. Pathology 1992; 24:37–39.

15. Cattaneo A, Bracco GL, Maestrini G, Carli P, Taddei GL, Calafranceschi M, Marchionni M. Lichen sclerosus and squamous hyperplasia of the vulva. A clinical study of medical treatment. J Reprod Med 1991; 36:301–305.

16. Cho D, Woodruff JD. Trichoepithelioma of the vulva. A report of two cases. J Reprod Med 1988; 33:317–319.

17. Christensen WN, Friedman KJ, Woodruff JD, Hood AF. Histologic characteristics of vulvar nevocellular nevi. J Cutan Pathol 1987; 14:87–91.

18. Cilla G, Pico F, Peris A, Idigoras P, Urbieta M, Perez-Trallero E. Human genital myiasis due to Sarcophaga. Rev Clin Esp 1992; 190:189–190.

19. Cockerell CJ, LeBoit PE. Bacillary angiomatosis: a newly characterized, pseudoneoplastic, infectious, cutaneous vascular disorder. J Am Acad Dermatol 1990; 22:501–512.

20. Cone R, Beckmann A, Aho M, Wahlstrom T, Ek M, Corey L, Paavonen J. Subclinical manifestations of vulvar human papillomavirus infection. Int J Gynecol Pathol 1991; 10:26–35.

21. Cooper PH. Acantholytic dermatosis localized to the vulvocrural area. J Cutan Pathol 1989; 16:81–84.

22. Corey L, Adams HG, Brown ZA, Holmes KK. Genital herpes simplex virus infections: clinical manifestations, course, and complications. Ann Intern Med 1983; 98:958.

23. Dalziel KL, Mallard R, Wojnarowska F. The treatment of vulvar lichen sclerosus with very potent topical steroid (clobetasol propionate 0.05% cream). Br J Dermatol 1991; 124:461.

24. Das SP. Paraurethral cysts in women. J Urol 1981; 126:41–43.

25. Degefu S, Dhurandhar N, O'Quinn AG, Fuller PN. Granular cell tumor of the clitoris in pregnancy. Gynecol Oncol 1984; 19:246.

26. Derksen DJ. Children with condylomata acuminata. J Fam Pract 1992; 34:419–423.

27. Dewhurst DJ. Congenital malformations of the genital tract in childhood. J Obstet Gynecol Br Commun 1968; 75:377.

28. Dodson RF, Fritz GS, Hubler WR, Rudolph AH, Knox JM, Chu LW. Donovanosis: a morphologic study. J Invest Dermatol 1974; 62:611.

29. Dunn JM. Congenital absence of the external genitalia. J Reprod Med 1970; 4:66.

30. Duray PH, Merino MJ, Axiotis C. Warty dyskeratoma of the vulva. Int J Gynecol Pathol 1983; 2:286.

31. Edwards L. Vulvar lichen planus. Arch Dermatol 1989; 125:1677–1680.

32. Edwards L. Desquamative vulvitis. Dermatol Clin 1992; 10:325–337.

33. Evron S, Leviatan A, Okon F. Familial benign chronic pemphigus appearing as leukoplakia of the vulva. Int J Dermatol 1984; 23:556.

34. Faber K, Jones MA, Spratt D, Tarraza HM, Jr. Vulvar leiomyomatosis in a patient with esophagogastric leiomyomatosis: review of the syndrome. Gynecol Oncol 1991; 41:92–94.

35. Falk HC, Hyman AB. Congenital absence of clitoris. Obstet Gynecol 1971; 38:269.

36. Ferenczy A, Mitao M, Nagai N, Silverstein SJ, Crum CP. Latent papillomavirus and recurring genital warts. N Engl J Med 1985; 313:784.

37. Fletcher CD, Tsang WY, Fisher C, Lee KC, Chan JK. Angiomyofibroblastoma of the vulva: a benign neoplasm distinct from aggressive angiomyxoma. Am J Surg Pathol 1992; 16:373–382.

38. Friedman RJ, Ackerman B. Difficulties in the histologic diagnosis of melanocytic nevi on the vulvae of premenopausal women, In: Ackerman AB, ed. Pathology of malignant melanoma. New York: Masson, 1981:119–127.

39. Freidmann W, Schafer A, Kretschmer R, CMV virus infection of the vulva and vagina. Geburtshilfe-Frauenheilkd 1990; 50:729–730.

40. Friedrich EG, Jr. Vulvar vestibulitis syndrome. J Reprod Med 1987; 32:110–114.

41. Friedrich EG, Jr, MacLaren NK. Genetic aspects of vulvar lichen sclerosus. Am J Obstet Gynecol 1984; 150:161.

42. Friedrich EG Jr, Burch K, Bahr JP. The vulvar clinic: an eight year appraisal. Am J Obstet Gynecol 1979; 135:1036.

43. Friedrich EG, Jr, Wilkinson EJ. Mucous cysts of the vulvar vestibule. Obstet Gynecol 1973; 42:407.

44. Friedrich EG, Jr, Wilkinson EJ. Vulvar surgery for neurofibromatosis. Obstet Gynecol 1985; 65:135.

45. Frith P, Charnock M, Wojnarowska F. Cicatricial pemphigoid diagnosed from ocular features in recurrent severe vulvae scarring. Two case reports. Br J Obstet Gynecol 1991; 98:482–484.

46. Fukamizu H, Matsumoto K, Inouek K, Moriguchi T. Large vulvar lipoma. Arch Dermatol 1982; 118:447.

47. Fukaya Y, Ueda H. A case of idiopathic vulvar calcinosis. The first in Japan. J Dermatol 1991; 18:680–683.

48. Gaffney EF, Majmuder B, Bryan JA. Nodular fasciitis (pseudosarcomatous fasciitis) of the vulva. Int J Gynecol Pathol 1982; 1:307.

49. Gilks CB, Clement PB, Wood WS. Trichoblastic fibroma. A clinicopathologic study of three cases. Am J Dermatopathol 1989; 11:397–402.

50. Growdon WA, Fu Y, Lebherz TB, Rapkin A, Mason GD, Parks G. Pruritic vulvar squamous papillomatosis: evidence for human papillomavirus etiology. Obstet Gynecol 1985; 66:564.

51. Hackel H, Hartmann AA, Burg G. Vulvitis granulomatosa and anoperineitis granulomatosa. Dermatologica 1991; 182:128–131.

52. Hendricks J, Wilkinson EJ. KI-67 expression in lichen sclerosus of the vulva. (in preparation)

53. Hewitt J. Lichen sclerosus. J Reprod Med 1986; 31:781.

54. Hewitt M, Barrow GI, Miller DC, Turk F, Turk S. Mites in the personal environment and their role in skin disorders. Br J Dermatol 1973; 89:401.

55. Hewitt AB. Behcet's disease. Br J Vener Dis 1971; 47:52.

56. Holmes RC, Black MM. The specific dermatoses of pregnancy. J Am Acad Dermatol 1983; 8:805–812.

57. Huang HJ, Yamabe T, Tagawa H. A solitary neurilemmoma of the clitoris. Gynecol Oncol 1983; 15:103–110.

58. Imperial R, Helwig EB. Angiokeratoma of the vulva. Obstet Gynecol 1967; 29:307.

59. Isaacson D, Turner ML. Localized vulvar syringomas. J Am Acad Dermatol 1979; 1:352.

60. Iversen T, Aas M. Lymph drainage from the vulva. Gynecol Oncol 1983; 16:179.

61. Johnson TL, Kennedy AW, Segal GH. Lymphangioma circumscriptum of the vulva. A report of two cases. J Reprod Med 1991; 36:808–812.

62. Junard TA, Thomas SM. Cysts of the vulva and vagina: a comparative study. Int J Gynecol Obstet 1981; 19:239.

63. Katz VL, Askin FB, Bosch BD. Glomus tumor of the vulva: a case report. Obstet Gynecol 1986; 67:43S–45S.

64. Kaufman RH, Faro S. Herpes genitalis: clinical features and treatment. Clin Obstet Gynecol 1985; 28:152.

65. Kaufman RH, Friedman K. Hemangioma of the clitoris confused with adrenogenital syndrome: case report. Plast Reconstruct Surg 1981; 62:452–454.

66. Kellogg ND, Parra JM. Linea vestibularis. Pediatrics 1991; 87:926–929.

67. Kernen JA, Morgan ML. Benign lymphoid hamartoma of the vulva. Obstet Gynecol 1970; 35:290.

68. Kfuri A, Rosenshein N, Dorfman H, Goldstein P. Desmoid tumor of the vulva. J Reprod Med 1981; 26:272.

69. King DF, Bustillo M, Broen EN, Hiros FM. Granular cell tumors of the vulva. A report of 3 cases. J Dermatol Surg Oncol 1979; 5:794.

70. Kohorn EI, Merino MJ, Goldenhersh M. Vulvar pain and dyspareunia due to glomus tumor. Obstet Gynecol 1986; 67:41S–42S.

71. Koranantakul O, Lekhakula A, Wansit R, Koranantakul Y. Cutaneous myiasis of vulva caused by the muscoid fly (Chrysomyia genus). Southeast Asian J Trop Med Public Health 1991; 22:458–460.

72. Koutsky LA, Stevens CE, Holmes KK, Ashley RL, Kiviat NB, Critchlow CW, Corey L. Underdiagnosis of genital herpes by current clinical and viral-isolation procedures. N Eng J Med 1992; 326:1533–1539.

73. Kovi J, Tillman RL, Lee SM. Malignant transformation of condyloma acuminatum: a light microscopic and ultrastructural study. Am J Clin Pathol 1974; 61:702.

74. Krantz KE. Innervation of the human vulva and vagina. Obstet Gynecol 1958; 12:382.

75. Kremer M, Nussenson E, Steinfeld M, Zuckerman P. Crohn's disease of the vulva. Am J Gastroenterol 1984; 79:376.

76. Kuberski T. Granuloma inguinale (Donovanosis). Sex Trans Dis 1980; 7:29.

77. Kucera PR, Glazer J. Hydrocele of the canal of Nuck: a report of four cases. J Reprod Med 1985; 30:439.

78. Kurman RJ, Potkul RK, Lancaster WD, Lewandowski G, Weck PR, Delgato G. Vulvar condylomas and squamous vistibular micropapilloma: differences in appearance and response to treatment. J Reprod Med 1990; 35:1019–1022.

79. Leibowitch M, Neill S, Pelisse M, Moyal-Baracco M. The epithelial changes associated with squamous cell carcinoma of the vulva. Br J Obstet Gynaecol 1990; 97:1135–1139.

80. LiVolsi VA, Brooks JJ. Soft tissue tumors of the vulva. In: Wilkinson EJ, ed. Contemporary issues in surgical pathology. Pathology of the vulva and vagina. New York: Churchill Livingstone, 1987; 9:209–238.

81. Loening-Baucke V. Lichen sclerosus et atrophicus in children. Am J Dis Child 1991; 145:1058–1061.

82. Lucky AW. Pigmentary abnormalities in genetic disorders. Dermatol Clin 1988; 6:193–197.

83. Lynch PJ. Condylomata acuminata (anogenital warts). Obstet Gynecol 1985; 28:152.

84. Maccato ML, Kaufman RH. Herpes genitalis. Dermatol Clin 1992; 10:415–422.

85. Magrine JR, Masterson BJ. Loxosceles reclusa spider bite: a consideration in the differential diagnosis of chronic, nonmalignant ulcers of the vulva. Am J Obstet Gynecol 1981; 140:343.

86. Mahmud N, Kusuda N, Ichenose S, Gyotoku Y, Nakajima H, Ishimaru T, Yamabew T. Needle aspiration biopsy of vulvar endometriosis. A case report. Acta Cytol 1992; 36:514–516.

87. Maize JC. Mucosal melanosis. Dermatol Clin 1988; 6:283–293.

88. Majmudar B, Hallden C. The relationship between juvenile laryngeal papillomatosis and maternal condylomata acuminata. J Reprod Med 1986; 31:804.

89. Majmudar B, Castellano PZ, Wilson RW, Siegel RJ. Granular cell tumors of the vulva. J Reprod Med 1990; 35:1008–1014.
90. Mann MS, Kaufman RH. Erosive lichen planus of the vulva. Clin Obstet Gynecol 1991; 34:605–613.
91. Mann MS, Kaufman RH, Brown D, Adam E. Vulvar vestibulitis: significant clinical variables and treatment outcome. Obstet Gynecol 1992; 79:122–125.
92. Marinoff SC, Turner MLC. Vulvar vestibulitis syndrome: an overview. Am J Obstet Gynecol 1991; 165:1228–1233.
93. Marquette GP, Su B, Woodruff JD. Introital adenosis associated with Stevens-Johnson Sydrome. Obstet Gynecol 1985; 66:143–145.
94. Marwah S, Bergman ML. Ectopic salivary gland in the vulva (choristoma): report of a case and review of the literature. Obstet Gynecol 1980; 56:389.
95. McKay M, Frankman O, Horowitz B, et al. Vulvar vestibulitis and vestibular papillomatosis. Report of the ISSVD committee on vulvodynia. J Reprod Med 1991; 36:413–415.
96. McKee PH, Wright E, Hutt MSR. Vulvar schistosomiasis. Clin Exp Dermatol 1983; 8:189.
97. McNeely TB. Angiokeratoma of the clitoris. Arch Pathol Lab Med 1992; 116:880–881.
98. Meister P, Buckmann FW, Konrad E. Nodular fasciitis. Analysis of 100 cases and review of the literature. Pathol Res Pract 1978;162:133.
99. Merlob P, Bahari C, Liban E, Reisner SH. Cysts of the female external genitalia in the newborn infant. Am J Obstet Gynecol1978; 132:607.
100. Moyal-Barracco M, Leibowitch M, Orth G. Vestibular papillae of the vulva. Lack of evidence for human papillomavirus etiology. Arch Dermatol 1990; 126:1594–1598.
101. Muller G, Jacobs PH, Moore NE. Scraping for human scabies. Arch Dermatol 1973; 107:70.
102. Nadji M, Ganjei P, Penneys NS, Morales AR. Immunohistochemistry of vulvar neoplasms: a brief review. Int J Gynecol Pathol 1984; 3:41.
103. Neill SM, Smith NP, Eady RA. Ulcerative sarcoidosis: a rare manifestation of a common disease. Clin Exp Dermatol 1984; 9:277.
104. Oberhofer TR, Back AE. Isolation and cultivation of Haemophilus ducreyi. J Clin Microbiol 1982; 15:625.
105. O'Duffy JD, Carney JA, Deodhar S. Behcet's disease. Ann Intern Med 1971; 75:561.
106. O'Hara MF, Page DL. Adenomas of the breast and ectopic breast under lactational influences. Hum Pathol 1985; 16:707–712.
107. Oi RH, Munn R. Mucous cysts of the vulvar vestibule Hum Pathol 1982; 13:584.
108. Olansky S. Serodiagnosis of syphilis. Med Clin North Am 1972; 56:1145.
109. Ordonez NG, Manning JT, Luna MA. Mixed tumor of the vulva: a report of two cases probably arising in Bartholin's gland. Cancer 1981; 48:181.
110. Oriel JD. Natural history of genital warts. Br J Vener Dis 1971; 47:1.
111. Parry-Jones E. Lymphatics of the vulva. J Obstet Gynecol Br Commun 1963; 70:751.
112. Patton LW, Elgart ML, Williams CM. Vulvar erythema and induration. Extraintestinal Crohn's disease of the vulva. ArchDermatol 1990; 126:1351–1354.
113. Pelosi G, Martignoni G, Bonetti F. Intraductal carcinoma of mammary-type apocrine epithelium arising within a papillary hidradenoma of the vulva. Report of a case and review of the literature. Arch Pathol Lab Med 1991; 115:1249–1254.
114. Pincus SH. Vulvar dermatoses and pruritus vulva. Dermatol Clin 1992; 10:297–308.
115. Pincus SH, Stadecker MJ. Vulvar dystrophies and noninfectious inflammatory conditions. In: Wilkinson EJ, ed. Contemporary issues in surgical pathology. Pathology of the vulva and vagina.New York: Churchill Livingstone, 1987; 9:11.
116. Plentl AA, Friedman EA. Lymphatic system of the female genitalia. Philadelphia: WB Saunders, 1971.
117. Portnoy J, Ahronheim GA, Ghibu F, Clecner B, Joncas JH. Recovery of Epstein-Barr virus from genital ulcers. N Engl J Med 1984;311:966.
118. Pyka RE, Wilkinson EJ, Friedrich EG, Jr, Croker BP. The histopathology of vulvar vestibulitis syndrome. Int J GynecolPathol 1988; 7:249–257.
119. Ramesh V, Iyengar B. Proliferating trichilemmal cysts over the vulva. Cutis 1990; 45:187–189.
120. Reed RJ. Neoplasms of the skin. In: Silverberg SG, ed. Principles and practice of surgical pathology, 2nd ed. New York: Churchill Livingstone, 1990: 193–254.
121. Reed RJ, Parkinson RP. The histogenesis of mollescum contagiosum. Am J Surg Pathol; 1977; 1:161.
122. Reed JA, Brigati DJ, Flynn SD, McNutt NS, Min K, Welch DF, Slater LN. Immunocytochemical identification of Rochalimaea henselae in bacillary (epithelioid) angiomatosis, parenchymal bacillary peliosis, and persistent fever with bacteremia. Am J Surg Pathol 1992; 16:650–657.
123. Rhatigan RM, Nuss RC. Keratoacanthoma of the vulva. Gynecol Oncol 1985; 21:118.
124. Rhodes AR, Mihm MC, Jr, Weinstock MA. Dysplastic melanocytic nevi. A reproducible histoligic definition emphasizing cellular morphology. Mod Pathol 1989; 2:306–319.
125. Robboy SJ, Ross JS, Prat J, Keh PC, Welch WR. Urogenital sinus origin of mucinous and ciliated cysts of the vulva. Obstet Gynecol 1978; 51:347.
126. Roberts W, Daly JW. Pseudosarcomatyous fasciitis of the vulva. Gynecol Oncol 1981; 11:383.
127. Rock B, Hood AF, Rock JA. Prospective study of vulvar nevi. J Am Acad Dermatol 1990; 22:104–106.
128. Rodke G, Friedrich EG, Jr, Wilkinson EJ. Malignant potential of mixed vulvar dystrophy (lichen sclerosus associated with squamous cell hyperplasia). J Reprod Med 1988; 33:545–550.
129. Rorat E, Ferenczy A, Richart RM. Human Bartholin gland, duct and duct cyst. Arch Pathol 1975; 99:367.
130. Rorat E, Wallach RC. Mixed tumors of the vulva: clinical outcome and pathology, Int J Gynecol Pathol 1984; 3:323.
131. Rosen T, Tschen JA, Ramsdell W, Moore J, Markham B. Granuloma inguinale. J Am Acad Dermatol 1984; 11:433.
132. Rudolph RE. Vulvar melanosis. J Am Acad Dermatol 1990; 23:982–984.
133. Salzman RS, Kraus SJ, Miller RG, Scottnek FO, Kleris GS. Chancroidal ulcers that are not chancroid. Arch Dermatol 1984; 120:636.
134. Sedlacek TV, Riva JM, Magen AB, Mangan CE, Cunnane MF. Vaginal and vulvar adenosis. An unsuspected side effect of CO_2 laser vaporization. J Reprod Med 1990; 35:995–1001.
135. Sehgal VN, Shyamprasad AL, Beohar PC. The histopathological diagnosis of donovanosis. Br J Vener Dis 1984; 60:45.
136. Sherman AL, Reid R. CO_2 laser for suppurative hidradenitis of the vulva. J Reprod Med 1991; 36:113–117.
137. Sison-Torre EQ, Ackerman AB. Melanosis of the vulva. Am J Dermatopathol 1985; 7S:51–60.
138. Slavin RE, Christie JD, Swedo J, Powell LC, Jr. Locally aggressive granular cell tumor causing priapism of the crus ofthe clitoris. A light and ultrastructural study, with observations concerning the pathogenesis of fibrosis of the corpus cavernosum in priapism. Am J Surg Pathol 1986; 10:497–507.
139. Sood M, Mandal AK, Ganesh K. Lymphangioma circumscriptum of the vulva. J Indian Med Assoc 1991; 89:262–263.
140. Souteyrand P, Wong E, MacDonald DM. Zoon's balanitis (balanitis circumscripta plasmacellularis). Br J Dermatol 1981; 105:195–199.

141. Stage AH, Humeniuk JM, Easley WK. Bullous pemphigoid of the vulva: a case report. Am J Obstet Gynecol 1984; 150:169.

142. Stenchever MA, McDivitt RW, Fisher JA. Leiomyoma of the clitoris. J Reprod Med 1973; 10:75.

143. Stephenson H, Dottors DJ, Katz V, Droegemueller W. Necrotizing fasciitis of the vulva. Am J Obstet Gynecol 1992; 166:1324–1327.

144. Sun T, Schwartz NS, Sewell C, Lieberman P, Gross S. Enterobius egg granuloma of the vulva and peritoneum: review of the literature. Am J Trop Med Hyg 1991; 45:249–253.

145. Sutton GP, Smirz LR, Clark DH, Bennett JE. Group B streptococcal necrotizing fasciitis arising from an episiotomy. Obstet Gynecol 1985; 66:733.

146. Tavassoli FA, Norris HJ. Smooth muscle tumors of the vulva. Obstet Gynecol 1979; 53:213–217.

147. Tham SN, Choong HL. Primary tuberculous chancre in a renal transplant patient. J Am Acad Dermatol 1992; 26:342–344.

148. Thomas R, Barnhill D, Bibro M, Hoskins W. Hidradenitis suppurativa: a case presentation and review of the literature. Obstet Gynecol 1985; 66:592.

149. Tuffnell D, Buchan PC. Crohn's disease of the vulva in childhood Br J Clin Pract 1991; (Summer) 45:159–160.

150. Turner ML, Marinoff SC. Pudendal neuralgia Am J Obstet Gynecol 1991; 165:1233–1236.

151. Umpierre SA, Kaufman RH, Adam E, Wood KV, Adler-Storth ZK. Human papillomavirus DNA in tissue biopsy specimens of vulvar vestibulitis patients treated with interferon. Obstet Gynecol 1992; 78:693–695.

152. Van der Putte SCJ. Anogenital "sweat" glands. Histology and pathology of a gland that may mimic mammary glands. Am J Dermatopathol 1991; 13:557–567.

153. Van der Putte SCJ. Mammary-like glands of the vulva and their disorders. Int J Gynecol Pathol. 1994, in press.

154. Van Joost TH, Faber WR, Manuel HR. Drug-induced anogenital cicatricial pemphigoid. Br J Dermatol 1980; 102:715.

155. Venter PF, Röhm GF, Slabber DF. Giant neurofibromas of the labia. Obstet Gynecol 1981; 57:128–130.

156. Verkauf BS, Von Thron J, O'Brien WF. Clitoral size in normal women. Obstet Gynecol 1992; 80:41–44.

157. Von Krogh G. Warts. Immunologic factors of prognostic significance. Int J Dermatol 1979; 18:195.

158. Wade TR, Ackerman AB. The effects of resin podophyllin on condyloma acuminatum. Am J Dermatopathol 1985; 6:109.

159. Wilkinson EJ, Normal histology and nomenclature of the vulva, and malignant neoplasms, including VIN. Dermatol Clin 1992; 10:283–296.

160. Wilkinson EJ, Guerrero E, Daniel R, Shah K, Stone IK, Hardt NS, Friedrich EG, Jr. Vulvar vestibulitis is rarely associated with human papillomavirus infection types 6, 11, 16 or 18. Int J Gynecol Pathol; in press.

161. Kent HL, Wisniewski PM. Interferon for vulvar vestibulitis, J Reprod Med 1990; 35:1138–1140.

162. Wojinarowska F. Chronis bullous disease of childhood. Semin Dermatol 1988; 7:58–65.

163. Wolber RA, Talerman A, Wilkinson EJ, Clement PB. Vulvar granular cell tumors with pseudocarcinomatous hyperplasia: a comparative analyss with well-differentiated squamous carcinoma. Int J Gynecol Pathol 1991; 10:59–66.

164. Woodworth H, Dockerty MB, Wilson BB, Pratt JH. Papillary hidradenoma of the vulva: a clinicopathologic study of 69 cases. Am J Obstet Gynecol 1971; 110:501.

165. Word B. Office treatment of cyst and abscess of Bartholin's gland duct. South Med J 1968; 61:514.

166. Work BA. Pyoderma gangrenosum of the perineum. Obstet Gynecol 1980; 55:126.

167. Young AW, Herman EW, Tovell HMM. Syringoma of the vulva: incidence, diagnosis, and cuse of pruritus. Obstet Gynecol 1980; 55:515.

168. Young AW, Wind RM, Tovell HMM. Lymphangioma of the vulva. NY State J Med 1980; 80:987.

169. Zur Hausen H, Gissman L, Schlehofer JR. Viruses in the etiology of human genital cancer. Prog Med Virol 1984; 30:170.

INDEX

Page numbers followed by ''*f*'' denote figures; those followed by ''*t*'' denote tables.